Stress Counseling

A Rational Emotive Behavior Approach

Albert Ellis

Jack Gordon

Michael Neenan

Stephen Palmer

 Springer Publishing Company

First published in 1997 by Cassell PLC.
American edition published in 1998 by
Springer Publishing Company
536 Broadway
New York, NY 10012

Cover design by Margaret Dunin
Acquisitions Editor: Bill Tucker
Production Editor: Louise Farkas

98 99 00 01 02/5 4 3 2 1

Library of Congress Cataloging-in-Publication Data

Stress counseling : a rational emotive behavior approach / Albert Ellis . . .
   [et al.].
        p.   cm.
     Includes bibliographical references and index.
     ISBN 0-8261-1163-7
     1. Stress management. 2. Rational-emotive psychotherapy.
   I. Ellis, Albert.
   RC455.4.S87S767 1997
   616.89'14—dc21   97-33641
                                                               CIP

Printed in the United States of America

Please note: this volume contains its original British spellings.

Contents

Preface

I am delighted to have Springer Publishing Company bring out the American edition of *Stress Counseling: A Rational Emotive Behavior Approach*. When I first created rational emotive behavior therapy (REBT) in January 1955, stress counseling was almost nonexistent. Hans Selye had written a few important articles and books on the concept of the stress syndrome in the 1940s and 1950s but had not devoted any considerable effort to explaining how counselors and psychotherapists could deal with it. Richard Lazarus's book, *Psychological Stress and the Coping Process*, did not appear until 1966. In the meantime, I had published several books and articles on REBT, beginning with my first book on the subject, *How to Live With a "Neurotic"* (1957). In 1961, I published two books with Dr. Robert A. Harper, *A Guide to Successful Marriage* and *A Guide to Rational Living*, both of which show readers how to cope with a good number of stressful situations in their love and marital lives and in their regular lives.

In several important respects, therefore, REBT has shown professionals in the field of counseling psychotherapy, as well as laypeople confronted with stressful situations in their personal lives, how to do counseling about the stressors that all humans seem to encounter in their regular lives. This is quite expectable, because I derived the basic, now famous, ABC theory of rational emotive behavior therapy and what to do about coping with stress from the ancient Asian philosophers, Confucius, Gautama Buddha, and Lao Tsu, and from the ancient Western philosophers, Epicurus, Epictetus, and Marcus Aurelius. All these thinkers saw, thousands of years ago, that most humans tend to cope rather badly with the stressors of their personal and mated lives but that they have the constructive abilities to cope in a much more efficient manner. I saw that the ancients were correct about this and showed in my first paper on rational emotive behavior therapy, at the American Psychological Association Convention in Chicago in 1956 that, if people understood how they largely created their own emotional disturbances about stressful situations—if they changed their irrational and self-defeating thinking in this respect to rational and self-helping thoughts, feeling, and behaviors—they could lead much more effective and happier existences.

Following up these ideas and practices that REBT started to use in the mid-1950s, I then began to write a whole series of other papers and books for counselors and for the general public and I and a number of other early writers on REBT applied it to sex, love, and marital situations, to situations that involve raising healthy children, to school situations, to work problems, and to many other kinds of situations in the 1950s and 1960s, and to many other kinds of human problems since that time.

Stephen Palmer and Jack Gordon, together with Michael Neenan, have also been applying rational emotive behavior therapy to stress counseling problems for the past decade. They have worked with a great many individuals in England and have developed several stress counseling techniques of their own. They asked me to write a book with them on stress counseling in the 1990s and I was very happy to collaborate with them. REBT now has an international following as shown in the afterword to this book. We have a very comprehensive training program in REBT at the Albert Ellis Institute in New York, and we also have training institutes in REBT in several other important regions in the United States. These are always listed in our latest catalog, which is issued twice a year.

I am delighted to be one of the main authors of this book, particularly because it has such an international flavor. REBT was the first of the now very popular cognitive and cognitive-behavior therapies. I pioneered REBT with my writings and teachings in the 1950s and 1960s; in the 1960s Aaron Beck, Donald Meichenbaum, Maxie C. Maultsby, Jr., Albert Bandura, Arnold Lazarus, and other leaders in the field of psychotherapy began to adopt and adapt rational emotive behavioral methods. Because of their outstanding work and the great amount of research and practice that has been done by rational emotive behavior therapists, it is highly probable that various forms of cognitive-behavior therapy (CBT) and rational behavior therapy are the most effective forms of therapy now used throughout the world.

I am, of course, very happy to see that REBT and CBT are becoming increasingly popular. I originally used them to help clients and other people cope effectively with anxiety and depression. Both these disturbed feelings, and the dysfunctional behavior to which they lead, are almost always related to people experiencing significant stressors in their relationships with others and in their work lives, and then feeling quite upset and acting against their own interests and the interests of the social group in which they choose to live. Very often, too, people experience severe anger and rage against others and act self-defeatingly and socially defeatingly in this respect. So what is called stress counseling in this book covers, we could easily say, a multitude of sins! People feel exceptionally stressed, because they are not getting what they really want in life or are getting what they really do not want, and then fairly quickly and often prolongedly react with dysfunctional feelings and behaviors. REBT, along with the teachings of many ancient and modern philosophers, and recently with contributions from a host of psychotherapists and counselors, suggests that it is not only the stressors of life to which people react badly, but to their own belief system about these stressors as well. REBT asserts that practically all humans have innate and acquired constructionist tendencies and are able to overcome the stressors of life and to create problem-solving solutions to them. But it also asserts that people have strong tendencies to overreact or underreact to these stressors, creating emotional and behavioral malfunctioning. REBT says that counselors and therapists can quickly discover what are the main dysfunctional beliefs of people who react badly to stress, and how these beliefs can be quickly disputed with a combination of thinking, feeling, and behavioral techniques. My English colleagues and I outline some of these main methods in this book and show how they can be applied with regular clients, with difficult clients, in occupational stress, and in group work. We describe clearly and briefly the material in this book so that REBT can be applied effectively by almost any counselor who learns our system and who applies herself or himself to using it. We hope that we have nicely succeeded in these respects.

Albert Ellis, Ph.D.
President
Albert Ellis Institute
New York, NY

CHAPTER 1

Stress: A Rational Emotive Behaviour Perspective

The last decade has been notable for a growing interest and emphasis on stress-related topics in both the public and academic media. In academic journals there has been a proliferation of published research on stress and related topics, and at the same time, the public media have been drawing attention to the effects of stress on personal health and well-being in general. Stress management training programmes have been introduced to business organizations concerned about absenteeism in the workforce and in helping employees to cope more effectively with the daily pressures and demands of their job. However, despite the continuing output of published research on stress and anti-stress therapies, stress counselling, as Wagenaar and La Forge observed, remains vague and imprecise.[1] Part of the difficulty in discussing effective treatment of stress stems from the lack of a consistent definition of stress. Stress is not always bad; in fact, some individuals – especially those in competitive sports – have found that a degree of stress-related arousal can enhance their performance, while a lack of it has the opposite effect.[2]

It seems, therefore, that in a stress counselling context we are really talking about the emotional and physiological distress experienced by a person exposed (1) to a series of interpersonal and environmental stressors perceived as demands that exceed the person's capabilities of coping with them, or (2) to an ongoing situation perceived as sufficiently threatening to overwhelm the person's resources for handling it. Since an accurate conceptual model of a problem is a prerequisite for the development of effective solutions, let us begin by clarifying what we mean by 'stress'.

Conceptualizing stress problems from a rational emotive behaviour perspective

What is stress? The answer, according to REBT, is to be found mainly in the way a person perceives, interprets and evaluates environmental and other kinds of stressors. In other words, stressful conditions rarely exist in their own right, but certain life situations or conditions may be experienced as stressful depending upon the perceptions and cognitions of those who are reacting to these conditions.[3]

This is not to say that there can never exist circumstances that are intrinsically 'stressful'. If, for example, a group of randomly selected individuals are hijacked by armed political thugs – so-called terrorists – and are deprived of sleep, food or water for an extended period of time, and subjected to various kinds of torture, such as beatings and non-stop interrogation, it is likely that just about all of them will experience a level of stress that exceeds their capacity to withstand it, and will at least partially crack under the strain. For some, the experience may even be fatal; others who manage to survive will live with disturbances such as anxiety, depression and suicidalness, often accompanied by various kinds of PTSD (post-traumatic stress disorder), such as cognitive intrusion and sleeplessness. In addition lowered levels of immune system regulation and increased levels of catecholamines following prolonged exposure to severe stressors can persist long after the chronic stressors have actually ended.[4]

Of course, strictly speaking, the Stimulus does not cause the Response directly but acts via the Organism to produce the Response. It is the particular biosocial makeup of humans that determines the (human) response. Other living creatures with different biologies would respond differently to the same set of life-threatening stressors than would a human.[5] Thus, strictly speaking, stress *per se*, unlike gravitation or molecules of carbon dioxide, has no independent existence of its own. As Klarreich notes, 'Events in the environment are not significant unless the person attributes significance to them and perceives them to be stressful'.[6]

Clinically, stress appears to exist only in the nervous systems of humans as a synthesis of certain physiological symptoms and disturbed negative cognitive, emotional and behavioural responses to events or situations which are perceived and evaluated as a threat to one's life or well-being to a degree that exceeds one's capacity to manage them effectively, either temporarily or permanently. Thus the three key elements in stress are perception, belief and ineffective management or behaviour.

In discussing how stress is conceptualized we wish to emphasize two points. First, as we previously pointed out, we are really talking about distress, since not all stress is distress. Some 'stressors' are actually viewed as 'exciting' and 'pleasurable'. Second, stress can take several forms; it is used to denote anxiety, panic, depression, anger and other disturbed emotional states together with maladaptive behaviours and various accompanying physiological reactions that may in turn become the focus of secondary disturbances (for example, anxiety about hypertension).

What triggers the experience of stress?

Stressors described as extremely life-threatening situations, such as those mentioned above, rarely occur in most people's experience. The most commonly occurring stressors are negative life events. In REBT a negative event may be defined as one that has the potential or actual ability to trigger a chain of cognitive and emotional reactions leading to adverse outcomes for the individual in terms of his or her physical and psychological health. Examples of both acute and chronic stressors include natural and technological disasters, violent crimes, bereavement, relationship breakups, various job stressors such as job loss and work-related pressures and failures, chronically bad housing and serious injury or illness. In addition to these, Ellis listed early traumas (beatings), rape, major life changes, a series of apparently never-ending troubles or noxious events, lack of leisure, general fatigue syndrome (GFS), a boring existence, and hypervigilance as stressors that people typically face during the course of their lives.[7] Biological stressors include hormonal or neurotransmitter dysfunction, physiological overload, chronic lack of sleep and various kinds of debilitating injuries. All of these are examples of negative life events or stressors.

Recognizing stress symptoms

Stress consists of disturbed psychological reactions usually accompanied by certain physiological components.

1. *Physiological* reactions of individuals to internal or external stressors tend to vary according to the individual's constitution.[8] These may vary from mild and relatively transient gastrointestinal sensations such as 'butterflies in the stomach' to more serious disorders. Typical disorders that develop or worsen as a direct result of relatively prolonged exposure to various stressors include hypertension, migraine and tension headaches, digestive system disorders and a number of other more serious complaints. The longer an individual suffers from stress, the worse the physiological disorders tend to become.

Chronic stress acts to maintain arousal of the autonomic nervous system (ANS), and the biochemical effects of continued arousal of the sympathetic component of the ANS cause a gradual breakdown of the weakest systems in the body. The physiological consequences of one particular chronic stressor, caregiving for family members with Alzheimer's disease, showed that chronic stress could have potentially irreversible damaging consequences on the general mental and physical health of older adults in the longer term.[9] Hypertension, diabetes, ulcers and a lowered efficiency of the immune system may follow as a consequence of prolonged and unrelieved exposure to stressors which overcome the individual's coping resources, and therefore are experienced as some form of stress. Thus, counselling and stress management can involve helping the person to deal with the stressors in life as well as the physiological consequences of exposure to chronic stressors.[10]

2. *Psychological* aspects of stress include feelings such as anxiety, depression, anger, guilt, hurt, morbid jealousy, shame, embarrassment and envy. These may be linked with various other responses that can include sensations, imagery, behaviours, cognitions and physical symptoms.[11] As we noted above, as well as being part of the stress syndrome, both the physiological and the initial psychological reactions to stress may react upon one another and therefore complicate the overall picture. These 'second order' disturbances will be considered in more detail later. For the moment it is important to remember that a person suffering from any one of the different kinds of psychological stress listed above may develop a stress-related physical illness. This in turn becomes yet another stressor for the person to cope with. The consequence is that the person feels even more stressed and debilitated and may simply give up trying to cope with the problem.

It is important to recognize and deal with second order disturbances, for, as Martin found in his review of stress in psychomatic medicine, a much better predictor of health and illness than life events or stressors *per se* is whether someone goes through a period of 'giving up'. Anxiety and depression about one's poor health will almost always have a negative effect by making both the physical and psychological conditions more difficult to treat. For the client, fear, anxiety, helplessness and panic simply make physical illness worse or more difficult to cope with. The inter-relationship between physical illness and emotional disturbance is important to bear in mind when dealing with stress as it has obvious implications for deciding the most appropriate kind of psychological approach to be used in the treatment of stress.[12]

The rational emotive behaviour approach to stress counselling

Rational emotive behaviour therapy (REBT), formerly known as rational emotive therapy (RET), is a theory of personality and a comprehensive approach to psycho-logical treatment that was developed by Albert Ellis, a clinical psychologist, in the 1950s. A key element of rational emotive behaviour therapy is the emphasis it places upon the cognitive element in self-defeating behaviour. At the same time, rational emotive behaviour theory maintains that cognition, feeling and behaviour are inter-related and interacting processes, and that all of these must be taken into account if treatment methods are to be effective.[13]

REBT states that our perceptions and evaluations of events in our environment largely determine how we respond emotionally and behaviourly to these events.[14] The core assumption of REBT is that what we label 'stress' or 'distress' is deter-mined not by the unpleasant events or 'stressors' that people experience in their lives, but mainly by their Irrational Beliefs about what they perceive is happening to them. Thus, when subjected to various environmental or interpersonal stressors or irritants, one set of individuals will see themselves pressured but will not feel stressed. Such people see themselves capable of coping adequately with difficult circumstances or adversities in their lives. By contrast, other individuals confronted with similar kinds of stressors feel highly aroused emotionally and physiologically, and cope poorly and inadequately with their situation.

The key issue, then, as Abrams and Ellis note, is: how does the environmental or interpersonal stressor become oppressive?[15] What causes the dysfunctional emotional and physical states symptomatic of stress? And what can be done to help people to reduce their levels of stress and to function in a healthier and more effec-tive manner? Biological stressors, such as those listed above, can obviously contribute to the experience of stress, and even predispose certain individuals to experience severe degrees of stress, as can virtually any of the other kinds of stres-sor. Since only on rare occasions is it possible or realistic to help a distressed client by eliminating the particular environmental stressor(s) supposedly causing the client's problem, we are left with one main possibility: the psychophysical condition of the distressed client had better become the focus of our attention.

One of the primary goals of rational emotive behaviour therapy is to show distressed clients (1) that the unfortunate events they experience in their lives do not by themselves cause their distress, although they may contribute to it; (2) that their distressed feelings and self-defeating behaviours arise from and are maintained by the distorted inferences and Irrational Beliefs they hold about the unfortunate acti-vating events in their lives; and (3) that surrendering their irrational cognitions and replacing them with more rational philosophies will help them to reduce or overcome their disturbed psychological and physiological states we call stress and to emote and behave in healthier, and more constructive, or self-helping ways.

In their discussion of the nature of the personality and behavioural variables that mediate individuals' ability to cope with stress, references were made to the results of work carried out by various researchers which seemed to suggest that a disposition to optimism, an 'easygoing' attitude to life, and relatively robust coping strategies can play a part in determining how well an individual reacts to the stressors encountered in daily life.[16] While we would not disagree that specific personality characteristics can influence individuals' ability to cope with stress, nevertheless we believe that these characteristics encourage people to create various kinds of irrational cognitions about the negative life events or stressors in their lives. Following Abrams and Ellis we shall use the term 'stress' throughout this book to represent the *result* of several kinds of irrational thinking.[17] Since it is a cornerstone of REBT theory that our feelings and behaviour are largely determined by the way we think, and that thinking, feeling and behaving are all interrelated, this basic feature of REBT will now become the focus of our attention. In our discussion so far we have stressed the importance of individuals' Irrational Beliefs as the causative factors in the creation of stress. Let us begin, therefore by making clear what we mean by 'rational' and 'irrational'.

Criteria of rationality and irrationality

Rationality is not defined in any absolute sense in rational emotive behaviour theory. Given that human beings tend to establish important goals and purposes, such as to survive and to be happy, and to actively strive to achieve their goals, rationality means that which helps people to achieve their basic goals and purposes. Rationality contains *three major criteria*:

(a)   pragmatic;
(b)   logical (nonabsolutist);
(c)   empirically consistent with reality.

Conversely, irrationality is defined as:

(a)   that which prevents people from achieving their basic goals and purposes;
(b)   is illogical (especially, dogmatic, and 'musturbatory');
(c)   is empirically inconsistent with reality.

The ABC model of emotional disturbance

The ABC model of emotional disturbance is an explanatory device used in REBT to facilitate an understanding of how stress (and other forms of emotional disturbance) are instigated or 'caused', not by unpleasant activating events or circumstances in our lives, but largely by the way we perceive and evaluate these events. In the course of stressing (or badly distressing) ourselves, we tend to perceive, think, feel and behave interactionally. The REBT model also points the way forward to showing how people experiencing stress can be helped to reduce their dysfunctional reactions, acquire a more rational or helpful outlook, and seek to develop practical solutions to their problems, by using a variety of cognitive, emotive and behavioural modification techniques within an overall conceptual framework.

In the REBT model, A stands for some perceived unpleasant Activating Event or a set of Activating Experiences which may be internal or external to the client. A may also include some of the client's inferences about, or interpretation of, the event – such as inferring that an unfortunate event or Adversity actually happened when it probably did not happen. These Activating Events may lie in the client's present, past or the anticipated future. In the context of stress, A stands for some kind of stressor or Adversity confronting the client which may be short term or chronic.

B stands for Beliefs. These are evaluative cognitions, *about* the Activating Events that happen to the client, and are either rigid or flexible. If a client's Belief is flexible and helpful it is called a *Rational Belief (RB)*. Flexible beliefs take the form of wishes, wants, desires and preferences. When your clients adhere to rational, flexible beliefs about the adversities, frustrations and unfortunate happenings in their lives, and do not elevate their rational wants or desires into dogmatic 'musts', 'shoulds' or 'ought tos', they tend to draw realistic conclusions from their rational premises (that is, their preferences, wishes, etc). These take the following forms:

1. *Non-extreme evaluations of badness*: Your clients will conclude 'It's bad, or unfortunate, but not awful, or terrible', when faced with a negative activating event or stressor.
2. *Show evidence of toleration*: Here, your clients will tend to reach conclusions such as 'I don't like what has happened to me, but I can bear it'.
3. *Acceptance of fallibility*: Clients who unconditionally accept themselves and others conclude 'I can accept myself and other people as fallible human beings who frequently fail and make mistakes, but who cannot legitimately be given some kind of single or overall global rating such as good or bad. Also, life conditions are complex, composed of many good, bad and neutral elements, and thus cannot be given a single rating such as as just or unjust, fair or unfair, good or bad.'
4. *Demonstrate flexible thinking towards the occurrence of events*: Clients tend to refrain from 'always or never' thinking. Instead they realize that few things can accurately be classed as 'always happening' or 'never happening'. It seems that most events in this world can be placed on a continuum from 'very likely to occur' or 'occurring very frequently', to 'very unlikely to occur' or 'occurring rarely'. (See note (a) on page 16.)

Conversely, when a belief is rigid or dogmatic, it is called an *Irrational Belief (IB)*.

When clients adhere strongly to rigid, dogmatic beliefs they tend to draw irrational conclusions such as:

1. *Awfulizing*: 'It's *awful* (meaning more than 100 per cent bad) when things do not turn out as I demand!'
2. *I-can't-stand-it-itis*: or low frustration tolerance. Clients mean 'I *can't bear it*, or I *can't endure this* when things are as bad as they are, and I cannot see myself ever being happy at all, or ever happy again'.
3. *Damnation*: Clients are excessively critical of themselves, others and life condi-

tions: 'Other people are no good for frustrating me.' 'The world is a rotten place for putting so many hassles and difficulties in my way!'
4. *Always and never thinking*: 'Things are *always* going to go badly for me, and I'll *never* win approval from people who are important to me no matter *what* I do!'

C in the ABC framework stands for the emotional and behavioural Consequences of the client's beliefs about **A**. **Cs** are basically of two kinds: the particular **Cs** that follow from clients' rigid *Irrational Beliefs* about negative **As** will be disturbed and are termed *unhealthy* negative consequences, while the **Cs** that follow from flexible *Rational Beliefs* about negative **As** tend to be nondisturbed and are termed *healthy* negative consequences.[18]

Unhealthy negative emotional components of the **C** are deemed unhealthy for one or more of the following reasons:

(a)   they lead clients to experience pain and discomfort;
(b)   they motivate the clients to engage in self-defeating behaviour;
(c)   they impede the client from taking the kind of actions necessary to achieve his or her goals.

By contrast, the particular **Cs** that follow from clients' *Rational Beliefs* about negative **As** are termed healthy negative consequences. Negative emotional components of the **C** are deemed healthy for the following reasons:

(a)   they alert the client to the fact that his or her goals are being blocked but they do not immobilize the client;
(b)   they motivate the client to take a constructive view of his or her situation;
(c)   they encourage the client to take action designed to help achieve his or her goals.

This distinction in REBT between healthy and unhealthy emotional and behavioural reactions to the various negative life events in clients' lives is important in the actual practice of REBT. In the case of stress the **C** is often organic or physical symptoms.[19] Here, let us also note that if **B** changes significantly, **C** usually also undergoes almost immediate vital changes. In other words, REBT maintains that clients' Irrational Beliefs (IBs) are a common cause of these negative, unhealthy feelings and maladaptive behaviours that collectively we label 'stress' or 'distress' and that clients can be helped – by changing their **Bs**, to bring about radically different *healthy* emotional and behavioural Consequences (such as remorse, concern or sadness, rather than unhealthy guilt, anxiety or depression) when faced with negative life events.[20]

Abrams and Ellis (1994) do not suggest that there is an invariable linear relationship between stress-related illnesses and Irrational Beliefs. Instead, they maintain that the prolonged arousal and emotional anguish that have been shown to be the prime cause of most stress-related illnesses often accompany the Irrational Beliefs people hold about their unfortunate conditions. The process by which clients' Irrational Beliefs lead to the psychophysiological disorders typical of stress follows closely the pattern of Selye's general adaption syndrome.

In other words, we begin with a negative life event – the **A**, which blocks a person's important interests, goals and values. The client evaluates this **A** as being in varying degrees 'bad' or 'dangerous' according to his or her Belief system. If the **Bs** are rational – 'This Activating Event is bad but I can live with it' – arousal of the autonomic nervous system (ANS) follows, but no great distress may occur. If the **Bs**, however, are irrational – 'This Adversity is *awful* and I can't stand it!' – the arousal of the ANS will tend to be worse, and to be prolonged. Then the weaker systems in the body may begin to break down, and the client may experience the typical psychophysiological symptoms of stress. Therefore, the client's Irrational Beliefs *about* his or her Adversities are important to change.

REBT shows clients how to identify and uproot their stress-creating Irrational Beliefs by Disputing them by means of a variety of cognitive, emotive and behavioural techniques and by replacing these IBs with more rational alternative Beliefs leading to healthier emotions and constructive behaviours. At the same time as they show clients how to minimize or eliminate their negative *unhealthy feelings* of stress and the dysfunctional physiological and maladaptive behavioural Consequences that accompany their burdensome or 'stressful' feelings (by Disputing their IBs), REBT practitioners encourage people to feel *strong healthy* negative *feelings*, such as sorrow, regret, annoyance and displeasure in response to negative life events or **As**. These feelings are judged healthy negative because, as previously explained, they encourage and motivate clients to change or ameliorate, where feasible, the unpleasant negative events or experiences in their lives – in other words their stressors – and to execute behaviour that is likely to enable them to cope successfully with these stressors and to reach their goal of better functioning and health.

Once clients are induced to reduce their Irrational Beliefs and replace them with Rational – that is, realistic, scientifically testable hypotheses about themselves and the world – they tend to experience healthier emotions and constructive behaviours and are less likely to get themselves into serious emotional difficulties in the future, even if the original stressors continue to be present in their lives.

The three Major Irrational Beliefs

In his earlier formulations of rational emotive therapy, Ellis identified twelve irrational ideas which from clinical observation seemed to lie at the root of most emotional disturbance. All of them consisted of some form of absolutism, commonly expressed in the form of unqualified demands, dictates or needs.[21] Later analysis showed that these twelve irrational ideas could be subsumed under three main headings and that each of these core IBs included an absolutist rigid should or must that people impose upon themselves and that cause them immense difficulties.[22] Although clients express their Irrational Beliefs in personally distinctive terms, their individual variations usually involve re-statements of three major Irrational Beliefs or 'musts':

1. 'I absolutely *must* perform well and/or win the love or approval of significant others or else I am an *inadequate worthless person*.'
2. 'You and other people *must* under all conditions and at all times be nice to me and treat me fairly or else *you* are a *rotten, horrible person*!'

3. 'Because it is preferable that I experience pleasure rather than pain, *conditions* under which I live absolutely *must* be comfortable, safe and advantageous or else the world is a rotten place, I *can't stand it*, and life is horrible and hardly worth living.'

Emotional and behavioural consequences of the three major IBs are these:

The first of these Major IBs often leads to anxiety, depression, shame and guilt. These may in turn lead to social withdrawal and drug abuse.

The second of these Major IBs tends to lead to anger and rage, which may be associated with acts of passive aggression and acts of violence.

The third of these Major IBs tends to lead to feelings of depression and hurt as well as problems of self-discipline, including procrastination and addictive behaviours.

These three important Irrational Beliefs constitute the main factors in what we term emotional/behavioural malfunctioning or stress. Therefore, unless distressed clients are shown how to recognize and uproot their irrational belief systems and replace them with reality-oriented philosophies, they are unlikely to acquire the healthier frame of mind that can enable them to take constructive steps to change or ameliorate the stressors – the difficult conditions under which they live – or to tolerate them if, for the time being, they cannot be changed.

The following example will attempt to illustrate the ABCs of stress and to show how easily one can make oneself feel moderately distressed when confronted with an unexpected stressor by allowing one's IBs a free rein. This example will also demonstrate how easily stress can be potentially harmful to close companions, as well as encouraging the stressed individual to overlook alternative, more constructive ways of dealing with the stressor situation.

In succeeding chapters we will treat in more detail such matters as assessment, treatment techniques and related issues.

AN EXAMPLE OF STRESS

We can illustrate the dynamics of REBT by means of the following real-life example.

John, a 35-year-old manager in a telecommunications company, decided to have a two-week vacation in Florida. Special circumstances had restricted his travel arrangements to one particular period of the year, and as a result, he was obliged to set specific travel dates for both the outward and return flights which could not be changed. Two days before his departure, a cousin of John's, who knew of his travel plans, telephoned him to ask a favour.

The cousin explained that his elderly mother, who was an aunt of John's through marriage, had arranged to pay an extended visit to some of her relatives who lived in Florida. Since his mother was not in good health and would not be able to cope with the hassles of making the trip on her own, and as she would be flying to the same airport in Florida, and was actually booked on the same plane as John, would John be kind enough to meet his aunt, help her with her luggage, and accompany her on the plane until she reached her destination? John's cousin assured him 'On arrival, Mother will be met by one of her sisters, and you will have no further responsibility for her'.

John was not greatly enthused by the idea, but as it was a family matter to some extent, he agreed to his cousin's request. He made one stipulation: since a train journey would be necessary to get both himself and his aunt to the departure airport, John would meet his aunt at the railway terminal at an early hour. There John would take charge of his aunt, and the early departure would allow them ample time to reach the airport where John wanted to spend at least two and a half hours relaxing before his flight was due to take off. Experience had taught John always to allow plenty of time for the almost inevitable hassles and delays that one encounters when travelling to international airports these days.

John's request was readily agreed, and at the pre-arranged time all three met up. A quick check revealed that everything the aunt needed for her trip seemingly was to hand – passport, tickets, currency. John and his aunt boarded the train, and duly arrived without a hitch at the airport where they were almost the first passengers to check in their luggage. Feeling pleased that things had gone so smoothly, John turned to his aunt to suggest that they find a place where she could relax over a coffee and read the morning papers while he went off to make an important phone call and to browse around the bookshops prior to entering the departure lounge. Before John could even utter a word, he could see from the sudden look of consternation on his aunt's face that something was amiss. 'My God!' she exclaimed, 'I've forgotten my heart pills!'

'You've *what*!' John exclaimed, utterly appalled, as the implications of this piece of news sunk in. 'I left the prescription on the kitchen table at home', his aunt explained. 'I meant to pick it up just as I was leaving to come to my son's, but in my excitement I clean forgot all about it. I must have my pills, I can't go without them! What are we going to do?'

What, indeed! John quickly turned over various possibilities in his mind, all of them impracticable. There was no way he could get hold of that prescription before take-off time. He could hardly go off to Florida on his own, leaving his aunt alone to fend for herself. The choice seemed to be: find some way of getting the pills his aunt required, or cancel the trip!

John found his aunt a place to sit down – she was already looking pretty agitated – while he set off to find a pharmacy where he could obtain the medication his aunt required. That seemed more sensible than dragging his aunt with him. He knew his aunt must never be hurried in any way, otherwise she would be at risk of a heart attack. John had little hope of getting his aunt's heart pills without a prescription. Pharmacies in Britain are licensed to sell non-prescription drugs over the counter on demand, but other drugs need a signed medical prescription. But it seemed worth a try; surely international airports would have the facilities to cope with medical emergencies, John reasoned. Eventually John located a pharmacy and returned to where his aunt was waiting. At this point, John felt slightly tense, but not stressed. Being basically optimistic, he hoped that this unexpected problem could be overcome. So, together John and his aunt set off to the pharmacy where his aunt explained her predicament to the assistant.

The assistant listened sympathetically as the aunt explained to him her predicament. 'I'm sorry', he said, 'We are not permitted to issue prescriptions at this branch. We have another branch in South Terminal where they might be able to help you. I suggest you go there!' South Terminal! 'Jesus Christ!' John swore to himself. How long would it take them to get to South Terminal and back, he wondered? Their departure was from here – North Terminal. If they had to make a trip to South Terminal and return to North Terminal, that could mean they might miss their flight! They might end up cancelling the flight anyway if they were unable to get hold of the goddamned heart pills!

John could now feel his anxiety level rising by the second. Also, he was beginning to feel angry, not so much at his aunt, although she was the direct cause of the problem. Rather, it was the conditions; in spite of all John's careful planning to arrive at the airport with time to spare, here he was in a situation where the outcome was thrown into uncertainty – and through no fault of his own!

Once more, John set off alone to find the point where people boarded the automated train that would take them to South Terminal. The concourse was now becoming busy and John almost collided with several people as he rushed around looking for the sign indicating the entrance to the automated train that would take him and his aunt to South Terminal, and cursing the airport designers for not making it easy to find! Meanwhile, John was feeling more and more anxious. All thought of having a nice easy time browsing round the shops, reading a magazine, and making a long phone call to a woman he'd promised to phone before leaving the country, had gone by the board. Time was slipping away and still he was no nearer a solution to their problem. In his disturbed state of mind John could see no way to resolve the dilemma in which he found himself. He could hardly abandon his aunt and go off on his own. He had undertaken an obligation to look after her, and it was quite obvious that she could not cope on her own. For better or for worse, he seemed stuck with her. After studying various direction indicators, John found what he was looking for. John ran back to where he had left his aunt, and hurried her towards the automated train entrance, as quickly as he felt was safe in her condition.

They missed the first train by a few seconds. Inwardly cursing the world in general for making life difficult, for being so 'unfair', and feeling aggrieved with his aunt for being so 'stupid' as to forget her heart pills, John kept glancing at his watch, unable to keep still as he saw the generous margin of time he had originally obtained being eroded minute by minute, with still no indication that he would end up with what they were looking for.

John was now feeling more stressed as he continued to damn the world for the predicament in which he found himself. Eventually he and his aunt arrived at South Terminal, where the problem of finding a pharmacy began all over again. Once more, John parked his aunt at a convenient spot and practically ran off pell-mell to locate the pharmacy he hoped would 'save' them. The realization that his trip would be cancelled in the event of his failing to acquire a supply of the essential pills did nothing to lower his anxiety level. John now felt really 'worked up'. In spite of all his careful planning to allow for the unexpected, here he was confronted with exactly the situation he had planned to avoid. 'I might as well not have bothered to arrive at the airport in plenty of time!' he said to himself.

At last, John located the pharmacy, and returned once more to collect his aunt. On arrival, they found that the pharmacy was full of people lining up to collect their prescriptions. John found someone in authority to whom his aunt explained her predicament. This fellow sounded helpful. Could she tell him what the dosage was that she required and was accustomed to using? There were two kinds of pill, he explained, and he had to be sure that he issued only the correct strength of pill, the kind she had been used to. For the second time that morning, John stared at his aunt in amazement as she admitted that she had no idea what strength her pills were.

That was the moment when John lost his 'cool'. 'Do you mean to say that you've been taking these pills for years and years and years and you don't even know what strength they are? Ye gods!' Ignoring his angry outburst, the assistant, not to be outdone, came back with 'Well, there are two kinds of pills and they each have a distinct colour. If I show you them would you be able to recognize the kind you've been taking from the colour?' 'Yes', replied John's aunt.

The assistant disappeared into the back of the shop and reappeared a few minutes later with two packets of heart pills. He opened the first pack and displayed the pills. They were not the colour John's aunt was familiar with. Then the other pack was opened for her to examine. 'Are these the ones?' queried the assistant. 'Yes that's them!' she exclaimed. 'Are you *sure*?' queried the assistant. 'Yes, I'm sure', John's aunt replied. 'Are you *absolutely* sure?' the assistant continued. 'Yes, I'm absolutely sure these are the ones', John's aunt affirmed. 'Well, I don't know if I can let you have two weeks' supply, but I think I can manage to let you have a week's supply; we are a little short of supplies at the moment, but just bear with me and I'll see what I can manage. You'll have to take your place in the queue as I have to attend to all these other people waiting in front of you first', said the assistant. John's temporary relief at securing eventually some of the pills his aunt needed was quickly extinguished by the sight of this large queue of people all lining up for prescriptions. Once more he expressed his anger: 'Why the hell do people leave these things to the last minute?' he fumed. 'If somebody has a medical condition, they *should* have enough sense to make sure that their medication is the *first* thing they should pack before they leave home! Think of all the inconvenience that would be avoided if only people would *think*!'

But the world seemed deaf to these pearls of wisdom. The line was moving slowly – almost *deliberately* slowly, it seemed to John, and time seemed to be rushing past now. There was nothing for it but to wait. So they waited – and waited. John kept looking at his watch. His level of frustration tolerance was now practically zero! Five minutes passed. Then ten. After fifteen minutes had passed, and John was feeling desperate about getting back to the North Terminal in time to catch his plane, the assistant appeared, triumphantly bearing two packs – a fortnight's supply – of the right heart pills!

Hardly stopping to thank the assistant, John grabbed the pills and practically propelled his aunt out of the pharmacy and towards the automated train entrance for the return journey to North Terminal. On arriving at the North Terminal, John ran to the nearest monitor screen to check the state of their flight.

At that moment he nearly had heart failure himself; opposite their flight number the screen displayed 'LAST CALL'! 'C'mon!' John shouted to his aunt. 'It's our last call!' Gathering up every piece of hand luggage his aunt was carrying and adding it to his own, John took his aunt's arm, and feeling his own heart pounding now, he literally marched her into the departure lounge, through the various passport, ticket check and security controls, and into the corridor leading to the departure gate, where they caught up with a few late stragglers making their way to join their flight. On the way, John saw out of the corner of his eye a row of unoccupied public telephones nearby. Dare he stop to make a very quick call to the woman friend to whom he'd promised a long call from the airport? A quick glance at his aunt convinced him not to even try. She was looking so agitated and breathless by now with all her dangerous exertions that if John had stopped to make a phone call, she might well have had a heart attack there and then! Besides, how could he explain over the phone in literally just a few seconds of conversation everything that had gone wrong that morning? Without even breaking step, John and his aunt pressed on, and at last were ushered to their seats in the plane. They'd made it!

Half an hour later, his tension and anxiety having subsided, John was able to think a little more rationally about exactly how he had made himself feel so stressed.

Using the ABC model

Using the above example we will demonstrate briefly at this stage how the ABC model is used to understand how people become stressed, while later chapters will provide a more detailed analysis of assessment and treatment of great stress.

Taking the example above, at point **A**, John learns that his aunt has arrived at the departure airport without her heart pills and that she cannot safely undertake the journey without an adequate supply of them. That is a fact.

Next, John infers that there probably will be some difficulty in obtaining a supply of the heart pills she has regularly been accustomed to using. He also infers that if the necessary pills cannot be obtained fairly soon, then his aunt will be unable to make the journey and she will be obliged to cancel her trip. In that event, John infers that he too will have to cancel his trip and thereby lose his holiday for that year. Observe how many inferences are drawn on the basis of one simple fact – namely, his aunt's forgetfulness in arranging to bring an adequate supply of her heart pills. In later chapters, we will demonstrate the importance of accurately assessing the 'critical A' – that part of your client's Activating Event that triggers the Irrational Belief(s) that largely lead to the disturbed responses we label stress.

At point **C** (emotional Consequences), John's feeling of stress was initially anxiety over the uncertainty of what would happen if he failed to obtain an emergency supply of his aunt's medication. Later, as the problem appeared to become more difficult to solve in the time he had available, his level of anxiety built up, and with it his anger, partly towards his aunt, but directed mainly at the difficult conditions he was trying to cope with.

If as REBT theory claims, this episode of forgotten medication and the unexpected problems it created contributed to but did not directly cause John's emotional Consequence (anxiety and anger), what did? The main answer is **B**. But precisely what Beliefs did John have at **B** to make him anxious and angry and panic about losing the plane?

First, he had a set of Rational Beliefs (RBs). These mainly consisted of something along the following lines: 'How annoying that my aunt has forgotten her heart pills! I had planned to do a number of things with my time before take-off, but since my aunt cannot sensibly continue her journey without her pills, I had better try to find her an emergency supply as soon as possible. I wish this inconvenience had not happened, especially since there is little time in which to resolve the problem. I realize that this won't be easy but there is no reason why it should be easy. If it's difficult, it's difficult. Too bad! So let me see what I can do to get an emergency supply of my aunt's medication as quickly as I can – to keep her going for a few days at least. However, if I fail, then I'll have to consider what other options we have.'

Why are these particular Beliefs rational? First, John expresses a wish that his aunt's mistake had not happened. He obviously had planned to carry out certain activities in the time he had allowed before take-off, a perfectly legitimate goal, and one that under 'normal' circumstances he would have achieved. But as bad luck would have it, events frustrated his plans. His subsequent feelings of annoyance and concern were appropriate and healthy under these circumstances, as was also his determination to do something about obtaining an emergency supply of the medication his aunt required to enable her to continue with her journey.

So long as John stayed rigorously with these Rational Beliefs (RBs) he would feel healthily (though negatively) annoyed and concerned. Furthermore, he would tend to act in a determined manner to obtain a temporary supply of the pills his aunt needed and to actively consider what alternative courses of action lay open to him should he be unsuccessful in that respect. He would not feel anxious, angry and panicked about failing to obtain medication and about the possibility of cancelling his flight. Why? Because these unhealthy feelings would stem from his Rational Beliefs *plus* a different set of cognitions, namely, his Irrational Beliefs about what was happening to him at **A**.

To summarize these last few points, we can see that Rational Beliefs are Beliefs that help people to cope with undesirable circumstances or negative life events, lead to their *healthy* emotional responses (such as concern, annoyance, sadness or regret) and motivate them to act in response to these negative **As** in ways that aid and abet their basic goals and values.

Conversely, Irrational Beliefs (IBs) consist of Beliefs that lead to *unhealthy* emotional responses to negative life events or undesirable circumstances (such as anxiety, anger, depression and shame) and that impede the fulfilment of one's goals and values.

Now, we know that John did, in fact, feel anxious, angry and panicked about the situation confronting him when he realized the implications of the fact that his aunt had forgotten her medication and could not continue her journey without it. We know that John had planned to do a number of things before his flight was due to take off. So what kind of Irrational Beliefs would we be looking for to explain why he found the fact of his aunt's forgotten medication so 'stressful'?

First, it looks like he was angry with his aunt for unwittingly disrupting his plans. However, anger was probably not the main reason for his disturbed feelings and behaviour. Suppose that his aunt had actually brought her pills with her but they had been lost in transit on her way to the airport through no fault of her own. Would John have felt angry towards his aunt in these circumstances?

Probably not, yet he would still have been faced with the same problem of finding an emergency replacement supply of his aunt's pills. Therefore, he probably would still be making himself disturbed by damning the situation for being so difficult and potentially disruptive of his holiday plans.

It is clear from John's description of his feelings at various stages in his search for an emergency replacement supply of his aunt's medication that he had a low tolerance of frustration. He had what we term Discomfort Disturbance – in this case, grandiose demands about life conditions. This type of disturbance is seen in situations requiring a fair amount of patience. For example, 'When I stand in line for some service, I *must* be served quickly because I *can't stand* delays in getting what I want!'

To create his Discomfort Disturbance, John would be holding an Irrational Belief about his frustrating situation, along the lines of: 'My aunt *should* have checked that she had her medication with her before setting off on her journey. Since she failed to do so, the problem of obtaining an alternative supply absolutely *must* be quickly and easily resolved, and it's horrible and terribly unfair if it isn't! I *can't stand* having my carefully prepared plans for a vacation disrupted and the world is *a rotten place* for allowing it to happen!'

John's Low Frustration Tolerance (LFT), anger, and depression did not merely stem from his strongly *desiring* less difficult conditions and intensely *disliking* the frustrations and difficulties he actually experienced. They more directly stem from his demanding and insisting that such difficult conditions *ought* not exist, *must* not exist, and that when they do exist, they *must* be capable of being resolved quickly and easily, and with the minimum of personal inconvenience to himself.

ELIMINATING SELF-CREATED STRESS

The alternative to Low Frustration Tolerance (LFT) and the emotional and behavioural problems it leads to is high tolerance of frustration, which comes about when clients surrender their IBs that create and maintain their LFT, and replace these IBs with rational alternative Beliefs. How do we help them achieve this? Mainly by showing them how to Dispute, at point **D**, the Irrational Beliefs (IBs) they keep telling themselves at **B**, about the negative Activating Experiences they encounter at **A**.

Disputing may be done with a number of cognitive, emotive and behavioural methods. In particular, REBT vigorously emphasizes cognitive restructuring of clients' self-defeating philosophies and shows people who over-react to life's 'stressful' conditions that they largely are responsible for their own exaggerated reactions. It emphasizes that they have much more ability than probably they realize to significantly change their unhelpful emotional Consequences (such as great distress) by modifying their ideas and attitudes about the various stressors in their lives through a combination of thinking, emotive and behavioural attacks on their dysfunctional thinking and acting. We will consider these methods in greater detail in the following chapter.

NOTES

1. Wagenaar and La Forge, 1994.
2. Ellis and Abrams, 1994.
3. Ellis, 1978, 1994a.

4. McKinnon, Weisse, Reynolds, Bowles and Baum, 1989.
5. Ellis, 1978, 1994a.
6. Klarreich, 1985.
7. Ellis, 1993c.
8. Abrams and Ellis, 1994.
9. Esterling, Kiecolt-Glaser, Bodnar and Glaser, 1994.
10. Palmer and Dryden, 1995.
11. Palmer, 1996; Palmer and Dryden, 1995.
12. Ellis and Abrahms, 1978; Martin, 1984.
13. Dryden and DiGiuseppe, 1990; Ellis, 1962, 1973, 1979a, 1988, 1990a, 1991a, 1994a, 1995a, 1996.
14. Ellis, 1962, 1977a, 1979a, 1991a, 1994a, 1996; Ellis and Dryden, 1987, 1990, 1991.
15. Abrams and Ellis, 1994.
16. Dolan, Sherwood and Light, 1992.
17. Abrams and Ellis, 1994.
18. Crawford and Ellis, 1989; Dryden, 1995b; Dryden and DiGiuseppe, 1990; Ellis, 1994a, 1996.
19. Abrams and Ellis, 1994.
20. Ellis, 1979a.
21. Ellis, 1962.
22. Dryden and Gordon, 1990b; Ellis, 1994a, 1995a, 1996; Ellis and Whiteley, 1979.

(a) In our experience, clients suffering from stress frequently use 'all and never' thinking. Although not derived from the basic musts, these absolutist musts tend to include or imply overgeneralizations such as 'always and never'.

CHAPTER 2
Assessment in Rational Emotive Behaviour Therapy

In this chapter we focus our attention on the REBT approach to assessment of client problems. Although standardized assessment instruments are used by therapists at The Albert Ellis Institute for Rational Emotive Behavior Therapy in New York and elsewhere, traditional assessment strategies in mental health are largely bypassed in favour of assessment strategies derived from REBT theory itself. The rationale behind this position and its advantages and disadvantages in terms of treatment effectiveness over traditional assessment models have been comprehensively outlined by Raymond DiGiuseppe.[1]

The use of personality data forms can often help therapists to assess which irrational ideas a client spontaneously endorses at the commencement of counselling, and also to suggest aspects of the client's life which may benefit from counselling later. However, REBT counsellors spend relatively little time at the outset on gathering background information on their clients. Instead, they usually aim to obtain an accurate description of their clients' major problem(s) as soon as is practicable and to break them down into their ABC components. This follows logically from REBT theory, which postulates that clients' disturbed emotions and behaviours largely stem from their faulty cognitions and irrational beliefs about the 'stressful' conditions in their lives. Assessment in REBT is thus treatment-orientated and is an ongoing process.

REBT takes its stance on the hypothetical–deductive, constructivist approach to knowledge.[2] Based on the philosophy of science advocated by philosophers and historians of science, REBT therapists formulate hypotheses concerning clients' diagnoses early in the interview, and then proceed to test their theories by logically deducing hypotheses and empirically testing them.[3] Popper has argued that it is important to deduce testable hypotheses from theories in a way that can be falsified. The importance of this notion of falsifiability lies in the fact that humans are often reluctant to abandon their constructed theories and hypotheses and prefer to stick with familiar ideas and shared paradigms. According to Popper, falsifiability is a main criterion of demarcation between science and non-science.[4]

Assessment is hypothesis-driven

Since assessment is, as we have stated, an ongoing process, diagnostic impressions are hypotheses and subject to change as new information comes to light during the counselling process. Ongoing assessment therefore provides a check on the effectiveness of the therapist's interventions and subsequently guides further clinical decisions. Therapists are encouraged to test their hypotheses as quickly as possible so as to arrive at the point where treatment decisions can be implemented. Since assessment is ongoing, therapists can construct questions to check whether their hypotheses about the client's problem are confirmed as tentatively true, and also to deduce other facts about the client's behaviour they would expect to discover if their hypotheses were true.

As DiGiuseppe pointed out, the most important aspects of assessment are those that lead to treatment decisions; these, in turn, need to be based on the latest and most relevant hypotheses concerning the nature of the client's problem.[5] Having at his or her command a theoretical knowledge base from which one can draw for ideas enables the therapist to quickly confirm or disconfirm earlier impressions and hypotheses and to develop new hypotheses if appropriate. Clients benefit by seeing how scientific thinking as modelled for them by the therapist clarifies the nature of their emotional and behavioural problems and points the way to their solution.

Ideally, the goal of counselling in rational emotive behaviour therapy is to encourage clients to make a profound philosophic change by learning how to apply the scientific method of thinking, when they are on their own, to any subsequent problems they may have both inside and outside the consulting room. The goal is for them to ultimately rarely distress themselves about virtually anything that can happen to them during the course of their lives. While not all clients achieve this goal, most clients are shown: (a) how to think more rationally, i.e. logically, realistically, scientifically about the negative events in their lives; (b) to emote more healthily to these negative events; and (c) to act more constructively to achieve their basic goals and purposes. If the therapist shows the client how to execute these tasks efficiently, the client perceives that the therapist is actively focusing on understanding his or her immediate problem and demonstrating a willingness and competence to deal with the client's pain. The client feels understood and will tend to disclose further important information to the therapist.[6]

Since therapists can, of course, be wrong about their interpretations, their frequently seeking feedback from the client on the accuracy of the therapist's interpretations helps to avoid the pursuit of irrelevant lines of enquiry and waste of therapeutic time. Also it does no harm to the therapeutic alliance if the client sees himself or herself as a collaborator with the therapist in the counselling process rather than a passive recipient of the therapist's interpretations.

DiGiuseppe recommends that to avoid giving the client the impression that the therapist has a closed mind about the client's problem and is unwilling to consider other possible interpretations, the therapist should offer interpretations in hypothetical language rather than in declarative sentences: 'Could it be true that you're feeling ...?' or 'I have an idea I would like to share with you. Is it possible that ...?'[7]

While REBT advocates that assessment focus on issues that are relevant to treatment, there are certain diagnostic categories – psychotic syndromes and biologically based depression, for example, that may best be treated with medication, after the therapist uses REBT and standard traditional assessment procedures. But even in these cases, patients may benefit from REBT concurrently with medication.[8] See Chapter 8 for a fuller discussion of these issues. We will now look in more detail at the basic sequence of assessment.

ASSESSMENT: THE BASIC SEQUENCE

As stated above, probably the best way to develop a therapeutic alliance is to try to identify and solve the client's immediate problem. Clients are asked what problem they want to discuss. This is called the target problem in REBT.

Since REBT is a problem-solving approach to psychotherapy, clients are encouraged to describe their problem as concretely as possible. As clients describe their problem the therapist intervenes fairly early – sometimes even in the first session, to break it down into its ABC components. Assessment of the As, the emotional consequences (Cs) and the IBs that give rise to the Cs is the main focus of the therapist's task at this stage and is usually the most efficient use of the therapist's time.

In addition to identifying the client's primary problem, it is important at this stage to identify and overcome any secondary problem the client may have about this problem. For example, a secondary problem (a problem about a problem) may exist when the client feels ashamed about feeling anxious, or guilty about feeling angry. If the existence of a secondary problem is seen as blocking the client's ability to focus on working constructively to resolve his or her primary problem, it may make therapeutic sense to tackle the secondary problem first.

During assessment, REBT therapists usually take a highly directive stance. They know from their theoretical knowledge and clinical experience what they are looking for. As the therapist's questioning elicits more and more information from the client, the therapist directs the client's attention to the C (the feelings he or she has about the A situation) and helps the client to identify whether he or she experienced a healthy negative feeling or an unhealthy feeling. Therapists need to be careful here to check that the client can distinguish accurately an unhealthy negative emotion from a healthy negative emotion and that the client and the therapist are working with a shared vocabulary. If this is not the case, confusion results, with the therapist and client working at cross purposes.

If the therapist's questioning reveals that the client reports experiencing an unhealthy negative emotion, the client's attention is then directed to the critical A. The critical A, as Dryden notes, is that aspect of the A that the client is most disturbed about.[9]

Once clients see that the therapist understands what they are feeling and thinking, and once they begin to accept the therapist's explanation of the ABC model that disturbed feelings largely stem from their Irrational Beliefs, the therapist can then proceed to assess these Irrational Beliefs. This is the most important diagnostic task in rational emotive behaviour therapy. In carrying it out, therapists need to be able to distinguish what Beck and his colleagues[10] term 'automatic thoughts', or what REBT theory refers to as inferences, on the one hand, and Irrational Beliefs, on the other.

It is important to realize that in assessing the **A** (Activating Event) for example, the therapist is not only trying to assess the objective situation confronting the client, but also the client's subjective perceptions of that situation. This means looking for the client's inferences about **A**, those personal interpretations that go beyond observable data but are personally significant to the client and that are likely to be implicated in the client's emotional experience. The therapist first assesses the actual and/or inferred **A** that the client is disturbed about at **C** (emotional Consequence). This includes identifying the relevant inference involved, the particular inference, or 'critical A', which triggered the client's Irrational Beliefs.[11]

While noting the client's negative inferences about the alleged source of their distressed feelings, REBT therapists may avoid challenging the validity of these inferences. Their aim at this stage may be to identify the most important **A** which triggered the client's Irrational Beliefs. We will now outline methods of identifying this important **A**.

Inference chaining

There are several ways of doing inference chaining about the **A**. Since a full description of all these methods is beyond the scope of this chapter, we will describe two methods that are typically used in REBT. Practitioners interested in a more extended treatment of inference chaining will find Dryden provides a comprehensive coverage of the subject.[12]

EXAMPLE 1

Therapist: What would you say is your major feeling when your wife gets home late from her bridge club?

Client: I feel anxious.

Therapist: Anxious about what? (Here the therapist has obtained **C** and is now probing for **A**.)

Client: Well, I wonder what she's doing. You see, it only takes her half an hour to drive the distance from the place where she plays bridge to her home. Yet, most nights she arrives home an hour later than if she got into her car and drove straight home immediately her bridge lessons are over.

Therapist: Have you asked her what she does during this extra hour after her bridge class is over?

Client: Well, I have. She says she stays behind to have a coffee and a chat with her friends.

Therapist: Is that a problem for you?

Client: Well, not exactly. (Client's answer hints that this is partly the problem, and that certain inferences may be involved.)

Therapist: Then exactly what is anxiety-provoking in your mind about your wife staying behind after class to chat and drink coffee with her friends? (Since the client seems to accept his wife's explanation but seems none too happy with it, the therapist probes for possible inferences the client may have about this.)

Client: Well, she might meet someone. My wife's a pretty attractive woman, you see. (Inference 1.)

Therapist: OK. Let's assume that other people – and particularly other men in the bridge club, find your wife attractive. What would you find anxiety-provoking about that? (Probing to see if inference 1 is relevant.)

Client: Well, she might meet some man who found her attractive and who might persuade her to leave me for him. (Inference 2.)

Therapist: And if she did? (Probing for the relevance of inference 2.)

Client: Then I'd be left on my own. (Inference 3.)

Therapist: And what would that mean to you? (Probing to see if inference 3 is the relevant **A**.)

Client: My God! That would be terrible! I couldn't stand that because I just know I could never find another woman as wonderful as my wife, and therefore I would never be happy again! (Irrational Belief.)

Having identified the client's Irrational Belief the therapist checks back to see which inference is the most relevant in the chain.

Therapist: What was most distressing for you about what you have told me? Was it:
  (a) your wife staying behind for coffee and a chat with her club friends instead of coming straight home after her bridge class was over?
  (b) the possibility of your wife meeting someone?
  (c) your wife meeting some man who found her attractive and persuading her to leave you for him?
  (d) being left on your own?

Client: Oh, definitely my wife leaving me for another man.

This example shows the importance of identifying the client's most relevant **A** and obtaining the client's confirmation that he or she perceives it that way. If the therapist had mistakenly thought that the client was mainly anxious about merely being left alone, she would have tended to look for an IB associated with fear of being alone. Identifying the client's IBs about his wife actually leaving him for another man and what her leaving would mean for the client, enabled the therapist to identify the most relevant **C** as depression. In effect, the client's anxiety served as a defence against the uncomfortable feelings of depression that would arise if the prospect of his wife leaving him for another man materialized. Notice how the client's **C** changed from anxiety at the commencement of the inference chaining to depression at the end of it. Such changes are not unusual when inference chaining is employed to identify the critical **A**. Not only can the **C** change, but sometimes the **A** too can change. When the therapist is confident that she has probably identified the client's most important **A** and verified her hypothesis about it she may proceed to Disputing of the appropriate target IB.

With regard to identifying the most important **A**, another method one can use in addition to asking the client to look at the inference chain and pick out that aspect of the chain that is the most relevant to his particular problem, is to vary some aspect of **A** and see how the client responds to it. For example, the therapist might ask the client 'Suppose that no males were ever present at your bridge club lessons, only females. Would that have had any impact on your anxiety concerning your wife's habit of staying behind for a coffee and a chat with her friends instead of returning home immediately her lessons were over?' If the client says he would not feel anxious in these circumstances, the therapist may be more confident that she is on the right track in her supposition that the client is anxious about the prospect of losing his wife if she socializes with other men.

Some cognitive therapists might prefer to challenge some of the client's negative inferences during the assessment phase. However, while REBT therapists may discover that the client's inferences are clearly distorted, they may often resist the temptation to dispute them. Instead, REBT therapists prefer to uncover and dispute as soon as possible the core Irrational Beliefs underlying the client's distorted inferences, particularly those underpinning the critical A. If clients succeed in giving up their IBs about their critical A, and replace these IBs with alternative rational beliefs about their A (including their inferences), they also tend to give up their distorted inferences.

Not all cases are as straightforward as the above example. Not only are inferences chained together but, as was shown in the example, two or more emotions may be linked together. Note, also, that a client's disturbed feelings at C may also serve as a second A leading to a new set of disturbances about his original upsetness – such as anxiety about anxiety, shame about depression, and so on. We refer to these as secondary disturbances or symptoms about symptoms. These issues will be treated in more detail in subsequent chapters. We will now describe a variation of inference chaining that is frequently performed by Albert Ellis.

Conjunctive phrasing

DiGiuseppe coined the term 'Conjunctive Phrasing' to describe the strategy Ellis uses when asking his client what she or he was thinking when she or he became upset. Sooner or later the client responds with an inference. Ellis responds to this inference, not by asking a question as in inference chaining, but with a conjunctive phrase. A typical response would be 'and then ...' or 'and that would mean ...' or 'and if that were true ...' or 'and that means I would be ...'.[13]

Observe that the conjunctive phrase does not dispute or challenge the inference. It assumes for the moment that the inference is true, and then, in effect invites clients to carry the inference through to its 'logical' conclusion – to 'finish their thought' in other words. As DiGiuseppe observes, 'An advantage of this method is that it keeps clients focussed on their thoughts. The less a therapist says, the less clients have to respond to the therapist's words or attend to whether the therapist has understood them. The conjunctive phrase focusses clients on the meaning of their statements. This strategy appears to be the most elegant and the most effective strategy for uncovering irrational beliefs.'[14]

To summarize, then, the purpose of inference chaining is to help the client to identify the most relevant part of the A. Next, the therapist assesses what the client's C now is about *this* A since either or both may have changed as was shown in example 1. The therapist then chooses whether to deal first with the client's anxiety about the prospect of losing his wife should she meet another man, or his depression if the new A were to actually happen.

Assessing A: pitfalls to avoid

First, discourage clients from providing too much detail about their A. Try to extract the salient theme or the major aspect of the A about which they are upset. Particularly voluble clients may begin to describe an A in great detail. As they do so, they trigger other thoughts about related issues and will often break off in the middle of a sentence and start to talk about some other issue before the therapist has had a chance to identify the first A. Allowing clients to jump back and forth between ideas that come into their head detracts from the problem-solving focus you are trying to establish. Tactfully interrupt the client and establish a specific focus on the main A: 'What was it about this situation that you felt most upset about?'

Second, discourage the client from talking about the A in vague terms. Your aim is to get as clear and specific a description of the A as you can. Once you get a specific A you can proceed to assess it using inference chaining if necessary to identify the most important A.

Third, work on one A at a time. This will usually be the one the client is most disturbed about. Make a note of any other As and explain that you will deal with them later.

Assessing the client's C

In the previous sections we focused on assessment of the A. You can, however, decide to assess the client's C before the A, depending upon which aspect of the target problem the client raises during the initial assessment process. When you undertake the assessment of C there are several important points to bear in mind.

First, make sure that you are dealing with an unhealthy negative emotion. In Chapter 1 we showed how to distinguish a healthy negative emotion from an unhealthy negative emotion. When making this distinction, it is important to ascertain that you and the client are using similar language when discussing emotions and that similar words have the same meaning for both of you. It is important to be consistent in your vocabulary throughout the counselling process.

Second, since a client's C can be an emotion or a behaviour, we would suggest that you often restrict C to denote an unhealthy negative emotion. This is because certain dysfunctional behaviours serve as defences to enable clients to avoid experiencing certain unhealthy negative emotions. For example, procrastination may help the client avoid tackling an important task if she or he would have performance anxiety when actually doing it. If the client mentions procrastination as a problem, encourage the client to identify the distorted *emotions* he or she would experience were he or she to refrain from procrastinating.

Assessing C: pitfalls to avoid

First, avoid the use of questions framed in language that suggests the 'A causes C' connection, such as: 'Did that make you angry?' A better way is: 'How did you feel about that?' or 'How do you feel about it now?'

Second, do not accept vague terms such as 'bad', 'stressed' and so on, when asking for your client's C. Clarify exactly what the client felt at C. If the client offers pseudo-feeling words such as 'trapped' or 'rejected' in response to your question 'How did you feel about ...' point out that there are no such feelings as 'trapped' or 'rejected'. Then ask: 'When you were rejected at point A, how did you feel at point C?' Try to ensure that your client's statements about emotions actually refer to emotions.

Assessing the client's IBs

Before you begin assessing your client's IBs try to see that the client understands why you are interested in identifying his Irrational Beliefs. In other words, see that your client understands that the emotional problem you and he have agreed is the target for change is determined by the client's belief and not by the activating event you have assessed as the critical A. If the client is not quite clear in his own mind about the B–C connection, it would be time well spent in teaching it until he demonstrates acceptance and understanding of this fundamental concept, otherwise he will fail to understand why you want to assess his beliefs.

Logically you can regard teaching the B–C connection as part of the assessment process. Several experienced REBT therapists have developed a number of exercises and metaphors to help teach the B–C in memorable ways, and these can be found in standard REBT texts.[15]

There are several important issues to keep in mind as you assess the client's IBs.

1. Remind the client of the distinction between rational (self-helping) and irrational (self-defeating) beliefs.
2. Assess all the components of the irrational beliefs, the dogmatic musts, shoulds, ought tos, followed by the four main derivatives: awfulizing, I-can't-stand-it-itis, damnation, and always and never thinking. While assessing the client's IBs, remind yourself of the three basic musts, or the three major Irrational Beliefs which we introduced in Chapter 1.
3. Carefully distinguish between absolute shoulds and conditional shoulds. Conditional shoulds refer to preferences and recommendations and do not account for clients' emotional problems. Help your client to distinguish between these different uses of 'should' or 'ought to' by means of examples drawn from everyday usage. Then reaffirm once more that disturbed emotions are created and maintained by absolutistic, dogmatic musts, shoulds and got tos. Again provide your client with examples of these and contrast them with the preferential and non-absolute variety to help him understand the difference.

USE QUESTIONS IN ASSESSING IRRATIONAL BELIEFS

Basically there are two types of question REBT therapists use in assessing clients' IBs.

The first is the open-ended question. A typical example in frequent use is: 'What were you telling yourself about A to make yourself disturbed at C?' The advantage of open-ended questions is that you are unlikely to put words into the client's mouth concerning his actual thoughts about A.

The disadvantage is that the client is unlikely to articulate an Irrational Belief without some didactic explanation of the basic principles of REBT. Once the client understands that his disturbed feelings arise from certain kinds of Irrational Beliefs he is more likely to come up with an answer to your open-ended question. You can then prompt him to search for his IBs by asking more open-ended questions along the lines of: 'Are you aware of what you were thinking at that moment?'; 'What was going through your mind then?' Even then your client is more likely to respond to your questions with inferences than to spontaneously come up with Irrational Beliefs in response to your questions.

An alternative to directing open-ended questions at A is to ask theory-driven questions. These are questions directly derived from REBT theory. For example, a therapist using a theory-driven question might ask the client: 'What *demand* were you making about your neighbour's disapproval of your behaviour to make yourself angry at A?' Another example of a theory-driven question designed to assess the presence of a derivative from a 'must' is: 'What kind of person did you think you were when you incurred your neighbour's disapproval?'

The theory-driven question has the advantage of pointing your client towards looking for his Irrational Beliefs. The danger is that you may be putting words into your client's mouth and suggesting that she holds Irrational Beliefs that she may not have. However, if you are fairly sure that your assessment of the client's C indicates the presence of an unhealthy negative emotion, that danger will be minimized.

Disputing Irrational Beliefs

Once you have completed your assessment of your client's problem and have clearly identified it in ABC terms, you can begin to Dispute your client's Irrational Beliefs. As you proceed, keep in mind your goals.

THE GOALS OF DISPUTING

The major goal of Disputing at the beginning stage of the REBT treatment process is to develop the conviction in your client's mind that his Irrational Beliefs are unproductive. This means helping the client to convince himself of two things: (a) that his IBs lead to self-defeating emotions and behaviours and that they are illogical and inconsistent with reality; and (b) that the rational alternatives to his IBs, that is, his RBs, are productive, make logical sense and are consistent with reality.

As you carry out the disputing process in relation to your client's problem, bear in mind that IBs consist of a primary must followed by four derivatives. These set the parameters of *what* you dispute. Thus you will be aiming to help your client understand the following basics:

1. *Musts*: There is no evidence to support the client's musts or demands but evidence can be found to support her preferences. Albert Ellis is often heard to tell clients 'There are most likely no absolute musts in the universe'. (In the following chapter where we look in detail at the counselling sequence, we will provide examples of teaching dialogues that REBT therapists have found helpful in conveying understanding of these basics to their clients.)
2. *Awfulizing*: When clients call something *awful* they destructively *define* it that

way. They are claiming: (a) It *must not* be as bad as it actually is; (b) it is as bad as it *could* be – 100 per cent bad; and (c) because it is *so* bad they can't be happy *at all*. They are, with this destructive definition, almost always making unfortunate Activating Events *worse* than they really are.

3. *I-can't-stand-it-itis*: Clients can in fact nearly always stand what they *think* they can't stand and *can* find some happiness even if bad events or circumstances at A persist.

4. *Damnation*: Damnation is a destructive concept in REBT because it is inconsistent with reality, is illogical and will lead clients into emotional trouble. People's *behaviour* may be deplorable but that doesn't make them *totally bad persons*. The rational alternative for clients is to accept themselves, other people and the world as fallible and complex – too complex to be given a single global rating.

5. *Always and never thinking*: It is most unlikely that a client will *always* be rejected, for example, or *never* succeed in doing well. No one is intrinsically unlovable nor a total failure.

We now turn our attention from the 'what' to dispute to the 'how'.

THE USE OF QUESTIONS DURING DISPUTING

First, focus on your client's must. Ask 'Why *must* you succeed?' It is quite likely that he will fail to answer the question you asked. Instead, the response you are likely to get will be along the lines of 'Because I want to!'; 'It's going to be well worth my while to succeed.' You can then point out to the client that he was not being asked why he *wanted* to succeed, meaning why it would be *preferable*, but why *must* he succeed?

The only correct answer to the question 'Why *must* you succeed?' is 'There is no reason why I must succeed although I would prefer to'. You may then educate the client, explain to him why his answer was incorrect, or why it was a correct answer to a different question. It may be necessary to use a combination of questions and didactic explanations until the client understands what the correct answer is and demonstrates his understanding by rightly answering a similar kind of question, e.g. 'Why *must* you get a good job?'

As an aid to facilitating client understanding of this basic point – the distinction between Rational and Irrational Beliefs – Dryden, and Dryden and DiGiuseppe advocate writing down the two questions:

1. Why must you succeed?
2. Why is it preferable but not essential for you to succeed?[16]

Ask the client to answer these two questions, reminding her where necessary of the distinction between IBs and RBs until she clearly sees that only the second of these two questions leads to a rational, productive answer.

Persist at disputing the client's absolutistic musts until the client – off his own bat, so to speak – can paraphrase Ellis's dictum, 'There are most likely no absolute "musts" in the universe'.

Having disputed the client's musts, you may then focus on some of the four derivatives from that premise (awfulizing, I-can't-stand-it-itis, damnation or always or never thinking). Persist until you have shown your client that there is no evidence in support of her musts before you begin to dispute one or more derivatives from them. If you switch from musts to derivatives, or vice versa, she may find this confusing rather than helpful. However, if your client does not find your anti-musturbatory disputing helpful, you may then dispute some derivatives of her musts and monitor her reactions. You may find that some clients find it easier to understand why the derivatives from their musts are irrational than why their musts themselves are irrational and untenable.

STRATEGIES FOR DISPUTING IRRATIONAL BELIEFS

There are three basic disputing strategies. The use of all three is likely to work better than focusing your attention on just one or two of them.

1. *Focus on illogicality:*   Your purpose here is to help your client to understand that his Irrational Belief makes no logical sense. Ask questions such as: 'Does it logically follow that …?' or 'Where is the logic?' Stress that your client's must about his pref-erence is magical: he magically believes that because he *prefers* something to happen that therefore it *must* happen.

2. *Focus on empiricism:*   Here your goal is to show your client that neither her musts nor the derivatives from these musts are empirically consistent with reality. Therefore use questions that ask your client to provide evidence in support of her Irrational Beliefs. For example, 'Where is the evidence that you must succeed? If there was some law of the universe that said that you must succeed, then how could you fail to succeed? Wouldn't you have to succeed irrespective of what transpired?' If your client is not succeeding at present, that fact constitutes evidence that her Irrational Belief that she must succeed is empirically inconsistent with reality.

3. *Focus on pragmatism:*   Show the client that his Irrational Beliefs simply don't work. They produce poor results for him. They will not help him to achieve his goals. It follows that as long as he clings to his Irrational Beliefs he is going to remain disturbed. Ask your client 'Where is believing that you *absolutely must* succeed going to get you other than anxious and depressed?'

Help your client to acquire alternative Rational Beliefs

Once you are satisfied that your client can successfully dispute her Irrational Beliefs and understand why they make no sense, help her to replace them with Rational Beliefs about her A. After you have helped her to construct RBs dispute them logi-cally, empirically and pragmatically. This helps your client appreciate that her Rational Beliefs *are* in fact rational, that they can stand up to critical examination. Your client had better convince herself that her new Rational Beliefs make sense, that there is evidence for them, rather than accept them merely because you have told her that they are rational and that they make sense.

USE A VARIETY OF DISPUTING STYLES

Among rational emotive behaviour therapists there are many individual variations of style in disputing clients' Irrational Beliefs. However, four basic styles comprise the basic skills of most experienced therapists. These four styles are Socratic, didactic, humorous and self-disclosing.

SOCRATIC STYLE

A therapist's main task in using the Socratic style is to direct questions at the illogical, empirically inconsistent and dysfunctional aspects of the client's Irrational Beliefs. The purpose of this style is to encourage the client to think for himself rather than to accept the therapist's viewpoint just because he speaks with some authority as a therapist. Experience shows, however, that even bright clients do not immediately catch on to the drift of their therapist's questions. Consequently Socratic questioning may need to be supplemented from time to time by the judicious use of short didactic explanations.

DIDACTIC STYLE

When asking questions in the Socratic style does not prove as productive as the therapist might hope, a shift to more didactic explanations may be more effective in getting across the idea that Rational Beliefs are more productive while Irrational Beliefs are self-defeating. Most therapists will, of course, use didactic style explanations with nearly all their clients at some point in the treatment process.

It is good teaching practice, when using didactic explanations, to check that the client has understood the point that you have been trying to get across to her. Thus you can say to the client 'I'm not quite sure if I'm making myself clear here. Would you like to put in your own words what you think I've been saying to you?' Also, do not accept without question your client's non-verbal signs of understanding (e.g. head nods, and other uncertain indications of assent) as evidence that your message has got through to your client. Test your assumptions!

HUMOROUS STYLE

With some clients therapists have found that a productive way of conveying to clients the idea that Irrational Beliefs lack supporting evidence is to use humour or humorous exaggeration. REBT therapists tend to be appropriately humorous with many of their clients since they think that much emotional disturbance stems from the fact that clients take themselves and their problems too seriously. They therefore strive to model for their clients the advantages of taking a serious but humorously ironic attitude to life.[17]

Dryden and Dryden and DiGiuseppe recommend that therapists use humour as a disputing strategy only if certain conditions have been met. These are if (a) you have established a good relationship with your client, (b) your client has already shown some evidence that he has a sense of humour, and (c) your humorous intervention is directed at the irrationality of the client's belief and not at the client as a person.

SELF-DISCLOSING STYLE

Using self-disclosure, you reveal that (a) you have experienced a problem similar to your client's, (b) you once held an Irrational Belief similar to your client's, and (c) you changed your Irrational Belief and no longer have the problem. However, some clients will not find this particular disputing style useful, and in certain circumstances it may not be in the best interests of the therapeutic relationship. In this case you may avoid self-disclosure as a disputing strategy and use other strategies such as those outlined above.

BE CREATIVE

Creativity can benefit many areas of life, and psychotherapy is no exception. We cannot tell you how to be creative; developing a creative style takes time. The more experience you gain in disputing Irrational Beliefs the more you will tend to build up a repertoire of stories, aphorisms and metaphors which experience has taught you can be useful in showing your clients in vivid or memorable ways why their Irrational Beliefs are indeed irrational and why rational alternatives will promote psychological health. This aspect of teaching clients the ABCs of REBT will be treated in more detail in the following chapters. We shall also include an illustration of the disputing process by taking as our prime example the case we described in Chapter 1 where John needlessly made himself anxious over the possibility of missing his holiday flight, and then made himself angry over the inefficient and time-consuming hassles he encountered at the airport when he tried to obtain emergency medication.

Summary

Rational Emotive Behaviour Therapy is based on a clear-cut theory of emotional health and disturbance, and the various techniques it employs in the assessment and treatment of emotional disturbance are used in the light of that theory. REBT practitioners believe in the therapeutic value of encouragement. They believe that it is only through hard work and practice that clients can make inroads into their long-standing Irrational Beliefs, replace them with more rational, realistic beliefs, and eventually help themselves to overcome their emotional and behavioural problems. Even when clients demonstrate intellectual acceptance of the basic principles of REBT and replace their earlier Irrational Beliefs with more rational alternatives, their new rational philosophy will sit lightly on their shoulders until therapists help them to deepen their convictions in their new philosophy. Long-held Irrational Beliefs, like long-standing bad habits, are tenacious. They don't just curl up and die overnight. Therefore hard work and practice lead clients to uproot their Irrational Beliefs and to keep disputing them until they cease to be a problem. That means convincing your clients that repeated rethinking and vigorous disputing of their Irrational Beliefs, together with repeated actions designed to weaken and undo them, will reduce and minimize them. Ways of achieving these goals will be detailed in the following chapters.

NOTES

1. DiGiuseppe, 1991.
2. Dryden, 1995a; Ellis, 1994a, 1995b.
3. Hempel, 1966; Kuhn, 1970; Lakatos, 1970; Popper, 1962.
4. Popper, 1962.
5. DiGiuseppe, 1991.
6. Dryden, 1990b; Ellis, 1985a; Ellis and Dryden, 1987.
7. DiGiuseppe, 1991.
8. Ellis, 1994a, 1995b, 1996.
9. Dryden, 1995a.
10. Beck, 1976; Beck and Emery, 1985; Beck, Rush, Shaw and Emery, 1979.
11. Dryden, 1995a.
12. Dryden, 1995a.
13. DiGiuseppe, 1991.
14. DiGiuseppe, 1991.
15. Dryden, 1987, 1995b; Ellis, 1985a, 1994a, 1996; Ellis and Dryden, 1996; Ellis and Velten, 1992; Walen, DiGiuseppe and Dryden, 1992.
16. Dryden, 1990b; Dryden and DiGiuseppe, 1990.
17. Dryden, 1987; Ellis, 1977a, 1977b.

CHAPTER 3

The Beginning Stage of Stress Counselling

In this chapter we focus on a number of pertinent issues that had better be considered before you begin counselling from a rational emotive behaviour perspective.

REBT is an active-directive form of counselling. This means that as practitioners you will be actively engaged in directing your clients to identify the philosophic source of their stress-related problems and in showing them how they can identify, challenge and change the Irrational Beliefs that largely create their disturbed emotions and behaviour.

Essentially, rational emotive behaviour counselling is a psychoeducational enterprise in which the role of the effective counsellor is conceptualized as that of an authoritative teacher who encourages and teaches his or her clients to learn how to become their own counsellor once formal therapy sessions have ended. In order to effectively carry out your role as a teacher of principles of rational living, you need to be conversant with a few recommended preliminary procedures of counselling practice, and to have a good grasp of several key elements of Rational Emotive Behaviour Theory. We will now focus first on the practical issues.

The therapist–client relationship

Rational emotive behaviour theory does not dogmatically insist on the necessity of any particular kind of client–therapist relationship; therapeutic flexibility is encouraged. Nevertheless, rational emotive behaviour therapists tend to think it desirable to establish certain therapeutic conditions and therapeutic styles with their clients to facilitate client progress.

THERAPEUTIC CONDITIONS

The three core therapeutic conditions that are important are (a) unconditional acceptance; (b) therapist genuineness or openness; (c) therapist empathy.

Taking each of these core conditions in order, REBT counsellors strive to unconditionally accept their clients as fallible human beings who frequently screw up but who are never essentially good or bad people no matter how obnoxiously or self-defeatingly they may behave in or outside of therapy. Unconditional acceptance of their clients allows therapists to evaluate their clients' thoughts and acts, but without rating the clients as humans in any way whatever.

In REBT therapists may bring to their clients' attention certain aspects of the clients' negative behaviour which is not in their best interests, but they especially avoid denigrating their clients for their negative or self-defeating behaviour. Also, by fully accepting themselves as fallible humans, rational emotive behaviour therapists not only act as good role models for their clients, but also help to establish a therapeutic relationship where both therapist and client can accept themselves and the other person as fallible.

Rational emotive behaviour therapists strive to be as open as is therapeutically desirable and do not refrain from disclosing personal information about themselves should their clients ask for it, unless the therapist has good reason to think that clients would misuse such information. The preferred therapeutic relationship is one in which clients see themselves as equal and active collaborators with their therapist in seeking to bring about fundamental change into their stress-filled lives, and where both participants see themselves as equal in their humanity, although unequal at the outset in therapeutic expertise and problem-solving skills.

By empathy, rational emotive behaviour therapists mean two things: first, they pursue the goal of offering clients affective empathy, i.e., communicating an understanding of how clients feel, and second, communicating to clients philosophic empathy, i.e., showing clients that they understand what they are thinking – see the philosophies that underlie, and give rise to, their feelings.

Given these conditions, clients can more readily accept their therapist as a highly active-directive teacher whose expertise in the psychology of human personality and its disturbances qualifies her as the one to take the lead in giving clients insights into the main causes of their problems, showing them how to come up with better solutions to these problems, and urging them to act on their new insights.

THERAPEUTIC STYLE

Throughout his long career as a rational emotive behaviour therapist, Ellis has consistently recommended counsellors to adopt an active-directive style with most clients. With clients who are exceptionally disturbed or resistant, he often recommends a particularly forceful version of that style.[1] Ellis believes that such a style, when introduced at the beginning of counselling, is important in that it helps and encourages clients quickly and efficiently to get to the philosophic core of their disturbed feelings and behaviours. However, other effective rational emotive behaviour therapists tend to vary their therapeutic style and may adopt a variety of styles to match the particular therapeutic requirements of different clients.[2]

It should be noted that the use of a confrontational style does not preclude the use of humour. As was shown in Chapter 2, humour may be employed appropriately by therapists when they wish to demonstrate to their clients in an empathic manner the sometimes amusing aspects of the latter's dogmatic Irrational Beliefs, and the therapeutic benefits to be obtained by taking a serious but not too serious view of life. However, not all clients benefit from the use of humour, so it should not be used if the client has already shown that he or she appears to lack a sense of humour.

If humour is used therapeutically, it is important that it is done within the spirit of unconditional acceptance of the client and that the humorous interventions are directed at the client's Irrational Beliefs and self-defeating feelings and actions, and not at the clients themselves. Here as elsewhere, therapists should try to be sufficiently flexible in their therapeutic approach so that they are able to vary their style of intervention to achieve their therapeutic goals and maximize their therapeutic relationships with specific clients.

An important caveat is in order at this point. Rational emotive behaviour therapists are advised to be wary of showing the great majority of their clients undue warmth in the counselling process. Exceptionally, depressed clients with suicidal tendencies may justify a distinctly higher degree of counsellor warmth than less disturbed clients, at least for a restricted period of time. Rational emotive behaviour theory maintains that if counsellors get really close to their clients and give them undue amounts of warmth, such as attention, caring and emotional support, in addition to unconditional acceptance, then these counsellors run two major risks.[3]

First, unusual therapist warmth may unwittingly reinforce their clients' dire need for love and approval – two Irrational Beliefs that rational emotive behaviour therapists believe lie at the core of much human disturbance. Clients appear to improve when this happens because their counsellors are in fact giving them the love and approval they believe they must have. As Ellis points out, these clients begin to 'feel better', but do not necessarily 'get better'.[4] Their apparent improvement may be illusory because not only may these clients fail to address the irrational philosophies which underpin their dire need for love and approval, but through receiving the therapist warmth they believe they need, they may actually reinforce their irrational ideas. Moreover, the fact of their clients feeling better as a result of their therapists' warmth may now interfere with the therapists identifying the clients' irrational ideas, showing them how these ideas relate to their problem and helping them to challenge and change them. Thus, although these clients may feel they have been helped by their counsellors, they have not been shown how to help themselves, and therefore remain vulnerable to future disturbance.

The second major risk is that therapist warmth may unwittingly reinforce their clients' philosophy of low frustration tolerance (LFT) – a major form of discomfort disturbance that many clients already cling to. The therapist's being warm towards the client is incompatible with actively encouraging, and in some cases actually pushing them, to involve themselves in uncomfortable experiences with the aim of achieving long-term therapeutic benefit.

As Ellis appropriately points out, clients with LFT problems 'almost always try to seek interminable help from others instead of coping with life's difficulties themselves. Any kind of therapy that does not specifically persuade them to stop their puerile whining, and to accept responsibility for their own happiness, tends to confirm their belief that others *must* help them.'[5]

A final point on therapeutic style: rational emotive behaviour theory is against insistence on absolute, dogmatic therapeutic rules. While an active-directive style is preferred for both theoretical and practical reasons, there may be occasions when your clinical judgement would suggest that a different approach might yield better results. Moreover, as we shall show in subsequent chapters, the relationship between counsellor and client tends to change during the process of rational emotive behaviour counselling, particularly with regard to the active-directive aspects of the counsellor's style.

At the outset the client usually does not have much insight into rational emotive behaviour concepts, and therefore the counsellor actively works to help the client to understand these concepts. As counselling proceeds and the counsellor receives evidence that the client does understand the basic concepts and is beginning to assume more responsibility for bringing about therapeutic change, the counsellor's level of directiveness decreases. When this occurs, the role of the counsellor becomes less directive and less prompting. The counsellor's role now focuses on encouraging the client to practise the elements of the rational emotive behaviour problem-solving method which they have been learning and increasingly using during both the early and middle stages of counselling.

To summarize, whatever personal nuances rational emotive behaviour therapists introduce into the therapeutic relationship or into their therapeutic style, their basic goal is to help their clients to identify the Irrational Beliefs that underpin their emotional disturbances and stress-related syndromes and change these beliefs in favour of rational beliefs. Once this is accomplished clients can lead more effective, less stress-filled lives, and learn to use these same methods to solve any future emotional problems that may arise.

We now focus on several important theoretical issues that rational emotive behaviour therapists need to be conversant with prior to engaging in the counselling process.

Biological bases of human irrationality and disturbance

In a seminal paper, Ellis hypothesized that all humans have a pronounced biologically-based tendency to think irrationally and become emotionally disturbed, as well as a similar tendency to think rationally.[6] REBT thus differs from other approaches to counselling – and is perhaps unique in this regard – in emphasizing the power of these biologically-based tendencies over the power of environmental conditions, including familial and cultural influences, to affect human happiness. But it by no means neglects the contribution of these environmental conditions to influence human emotion and behaviour.

The view that irrational thinking is largely determined by biological factors, although always interacting with influential environmental conditions, has considerable support. In his chapter entitled 'Fundamentals of Rational Emotive Behaviour Therapy for the 1990s', Ellis lists several reasons why irrational thinking, including absolutist musts, erroneous attributions, inferences and overgeneralizations, seems to be ubiquitous throughout human society.[7] The significance for REBT practitioners of the biological basis of much human disturbance – which is exacerbated by the influence of social and family unbringing – is that it helps to explain why it is difficult for people to make real and lasting changes, and why practitioners had better explain this to their clients, and to encourage them to keep working and practising to improve and maintain their improvements.[8] While we cannot do anything just yet to alter our biology, rational emotive behaviour practitioners can help their clients by emphasizing their other biologically-based tendency to think rationally and to use their reasoning powers to push themselves to work towards minimizing, although probably not eradicating, the impact of their tendency to think irrationally and the self-created difficulties that result from it.

Acquisition and perpetuation of psychological disturbance

Rational emotive behaviour theory does not put forward an elaborate account of the way in which we humans acquire psychological disturbance. This arises from the view discussed in the previous section that we have a biological tendency to think irrationally. However, rational emotive behaviour theory does acknowledge that environmental variables – especially social influences and family upbringing – do contribute to our tendency to make ourselves disturbed by our Irrational Beliefs.

A particularly significant point stressed in rational emotive behaviour theory is that humans vary in their disturbability. Children reared in dysfunctional families may be more prone to display psychological disturbance in later life than children reared in more favourable conditions, but this is not invariably the case. Some children who have been raised in harsh conditions display a remarkable resilience and in later life appear to display fewer signs of maladaptive behaviour than children who were well treated by their parents and brought up in relatively comfortable conditions.

Briefly, the rational emotive behaviour view of how we humans acquire our disturbed states can be partly summarized by the saying attributed to the Greek philosopher Epictetus: 'We are disturbed not by things but by the views that we take of them.' Or, in more formal language, we are not made disturbed simply by our experiences; rather we bring our ability to disturb ourselves to these experiences.

Rational emotive behaviour theory does, however, posit a more elaborate account of how we perpetuate our emotional disturbance. First, it argues that we do so because we lack three important insights. Let us describe these more fully:

INSIGHT NO. 1

Our self-defeating behaviour is usually related to Antecedent Events (**As**) or Adversities that block our goals and interests. However, these antecedent events do not, by themselves, cause our problems, but rather our Irrational Beliefs *about* these **As**.

As we teach our clients, 'You feel as you think, and your feelings, your behaviour and your thinking are all interrelated. External events, such as being mistreated or criticized when you were young, may have contributed to your emotional and subsequent behavioural reactions, but in themselves they did not *cause* your reactions. In the main, you create your feelings by the way you think about and evaluate whatever you perceive is happening to you.'

INSIGHT NO. 2

This is the understanding that regardless of how your clients upset themselves in the past, they are *now* disturbed because they *still believe* the irrational ideas with which they created their original disturbed feelings. They are still *actively reindoctrinating* themselves with these destructive beliefs – not because they were previously 'conditioned' to hold them and now do so 'automatically', but because they are continually reinforcing these ideas by their unhealthy actions or inaction, as well as by their unrealistic thinking.

In other words, it is clients' currently active – though sometimes unconscious – self-propagandization that maintains their disturbed emotions and behaviour and that enables these to disrupt their life in the present. Until they clearly accept responsibility for their still holding – and sometimes reinventing – these Irrational Beliefs, they are likely to make only feeble attempts to minimize them.

INSIGHT NO. 3

This is the clear realization and unflinching acknowledgement by clients that since it is their own human tendency to think crookedly that largely created emotional problems in the past, and that since they have persisted in disturbing themselves because of continued self-indoctrination in the present, they had better *work and practise* to change their Irrational Beliefs and self-defeating behaviours if they are to reduce them to a point where they cease to be a serious problem. Repeated rethinking and disputing of Irrational Beliefs, together with repeated actions designed to undo them, are required if these Beliefs are to be extinguished or minimized.

In addition to our lacking the three major insights just outlined, rational emotive behaviour theory contends that a second reason why we perpetuate our psychological problems is our adherence to a philosophy of low frustration tolerance. We tend to be short-range hedonists or seekers after instant gratification, and to believe that we *cannot stand* discomfort. We refuse to make ourselves uncomfortable in the present so that we can become comfortable later. We procrastinate by avoiding tackling problems which entail moderate discomfort, then discover later that we make these problems more difficult and uncomfortable than they were originally.

Clients who poorly tolerate frustration and discomfort frequently resist change even when they presumably want to effect it because of their proneness, which is both innate and acquired, to think and act against their own and society's best interests.

A third major way in which we perpetuate our psychological disturbances is the tendency of almost all humans to often create secondary as well as primary symptoms of disturbance. Thus, clients often make themselves anxious about their anxiety, guilty about their anger, depressed about their depression, ashamed about their embarrassment, and so on. In such cases, Ellis notes 'Although their [clients'] primary disturbances often have profound emotional, behavioural and cognitive sources, their secondary disturbances are perhaps even more cognitive because clients *observe* their primary disturbed feelings, *think* negatively about them, and *conclude* awfulizingly about their presence and continuance'.[9]

A fourth major way in which we perpetuate our psychological disturbances is our tendency to employ defences to ward off threats to our ego and to our level of comfort. We defensively deny that we have psychological problems when we definitely do. We refrain from taking personal responsibility for our problems, and blame either others or life conditions for our problem. When this happens in counselling, such clients tend to resist the basic message of the rational emotive behaviour approach, namely, that they *make themselves* disturbed – because if they were to admit this responsibility they might well severely condemn themselves. Unless the ideas that underlie their defensiveness are uncovered and dealt with, little progress will probably result.

A fifth way in which we perpetuate our own problems is by finding some kind of pay-off for having them. Thus, if we are having psychological problems we may therefore receive a lot of attention from others which we are loath to do without. We may see our problems as protecting us from having more severe problems.

When a person receives some kind of pay-off for having a psychological problem, she may be reluctant to work to overcome her problem because she may fear that she might lose the neurotic gain which she demands. When she sees her psychological problem as protecting her from a worse problem, she will not feel motivated to give up the existing emotional problem unless she can also be helped to deal with the 'worse' one she may encounter.

A woman may, for example, express a desire to become more assertive towards her domineering mother but balk at acting assertively because she fears she will be called 'bossy' and 'too big for your boots' and will be accused of being 'selfish' and 'uncaring' towards her mother. Clients may also become so habituated to their problems that they prefer to live indefinitely with a low but bearable level of discomfort than to undertake the more acute short-term discomfort needed to effect the rewards of long-term change. Such clients are said to be in the 'Comfort Trap'.[10]

Rational emotive behaviour theory holds that people adopt neurotic pay-offs because they make inferences and evaluations about the consequences, or likely consequences, of their behaviour. They are not directly influenced by these consequences.[11] You had better carefully assess self-defeating pay-offs if you want to implement productive therapeutic strategies.

Finally, we often perpetuate our own problems because we make self-fulfilling prophecies. Thus, a man who has difficulties in trusting women may, when he meets a new woman, be quite suspicious of her and indirectly discourage her from having warm intimate feelings towards him. This may lead to her leaving him and 'confirm' in his mind his original idea that women are not to be trusted. Unless you help clients who make self-fulfilling prophecies to see the contributions that they themselves make to these prophecies, they are likely to persist in perpetuating their problems.

Theory of therapeutic change

The rational emotive behaviour theory of therapeutic change states that if clients are to overcome the emotional and behavioural problems symptomatic of their stress, they had better carry out the following steps:

(a) recognize and acknowledge that they have a problem;
(b) look for and overcome any secondary disturbance about the primary problem;
(c) identify Irrational Beliefs that underpin their problems;
(d) understand why their Irrational Beliefs are, in fact, irrational, i.e., *illogical, inconsistent with reality* and giving them *poor results* in life;

(e)   realize why uprooting their magical, unsupportable beliefs and replacing them with rational, realistic alternatives will give them more productive results;
(f)   continue to challenge and Dispute their Irrational Beliefs until they no longer are convincing, and thereby strengthen their new rational philosophies;
(g)   use a variety of cognitive, emotive, imaginal and behavioural assignments to strengthen their new rational philosophies;
(h)   identify and overcome obstacles to therapeutic change using the same sequence just noted above, while still accepting themselves unconditionally with their tendency to construct such obstacles;
(i)   keep working for the rest of their lives against their tendency to think and act irrationally so that they rarely indulge in it.

Psychological interactionism

Rational emotive behaviour theory states that a person's thoughts, emotions and actions cannot be treated separately from one another. Rather, they are best conceptualized as being overlapping and interacting psychological processes. This is the principle of psychological interactionism. For example, when you think about something, you also tend to have an emotional reaction towards it and also a tendency to act towards it in some way. Equally, if you have a feeling about some person then you are likely to have some thoughts about her, as well as a tendency to act in a relation to that person in a certain manner. Similarly, if you act in a certain way towards her, your action is based on the way you think and feel about her, and it also influences your thoughts and feelings.

While REBT is best known for the emphasis it places on cognition, and while it is true that REBT emphasizes the power of thinking to influence human happiness and disturbance, it fully acknowledges people's feelings and actions, and their complex interactions with their thoughts. Therefore, rational emotive behaviour practitioners frequently use emotive, evocative and behavioural methods to encourage clients to change their thinking and acquire a more rational outlook on themselves and the world.

Moreover, REBT therapists are seldom just interested in symptom removal. Instead, the therapist aims to help the client to examine and change some of his most basic values or core schemas, particularly those which have caused the client trouble in the past, and are likely to make him disturbance-prone in the future.

Suppose, for example, a client has a serious fear of failing on his job. The rational emotive behaviour therapist would not be content to merely help him or her to overcome that particular fear, and to be less afraid in future of failing vocationally. Instead, he would be helped to give up exaggerated fears of failing at *anything* and shown how to *generally* minimize his basic awfulizing tendencies. The usual goal of REBT in stress counselling is not only to eliminate the client's presenting symptoms, but also to minimize many of her other (reported and non-reported) symptom-creating tendencies. In short, REBT strives for the most elegant solution possible to the problem of emotional disturbance and is seldom content with palliative solutions.

Rational emotive behaviour therapists define an elegant change as achieving a *profound philosophic change*. In order to help clients achieve this kind of elegant solution, REBT therapists employ not only cognitive techniques to dismantle their clients' magical, empirically unvalidatable thinking, but also a whole variety of behaviour modifying techniques adapted from existential, humanistic, eclectic and other therapies. These include role-playing, assertion training, desensitization, operant conditioning, and a number of emotive techniques, such as shame-attacking exercises, rational emotive imagery and humour.

Clients are shown how to achieve a profound change by working hard and persistently to have strong preferences instead of grandiose demands about themselves, about other people and about life conditions. They also had better see that making an elegant change requires something of a lifelong commitment and dedication to acquiring, reconstructing and steadily implementing an enthusiastic self-helping attitude.[12]

We can conclude this section by briefly summarizing the main points of rational emotive behaviour personality theory:

1. Human beings are born with a distinct proneness to create their own emotional disturbances. They also learn to exacerbate that proneness through social and cultural conditioning.
2. Humans have the ability to clearly understand how they originally acquired and have continued to maintain their emotional and dysfunctional behaviour, and to train themselves to change their self-defeating beliefs and habits.
3. Self-reconditioning requires self-discipline (which we can acquire) plus hard work and practice at understanding, contradicting and acting against people's irrational belief systems.
4. We tend to perceive, think, feel and behave interactionally. To understand and reduce emotional disturbance and needless distress, we had better use a variety of cognitive, emotive and behaviour-modification methods within an overall conceptual framework. In REBT this framework is called the ABC model of human disturbance. Clearly explain this model to your clients so that they understand REBT's effective counselling process.

THE RATIONAL EMOTIVE BEHAVIOUR COUNSELLING SEQUENCE

Preliminary considerations

REBT can be seen as a psychoeducational form of psychotherapy, with you acting as an encouraging teacher helping your students to grow by thinking for themselves. You encourage clients to question their own beliefs in an open-ended manner, to help them understand that their irrational beliefs are unrealistic, illogical and unproductive. Preferably, you show them how to use REBT to solve their emotional and practical problems throughout the rest of their lives. Using a hardheaded scientific outlook on the process of therapeutic change, you actively dissuade clients from believing in quick, painless and effortless 'cures'. Instead, you show them that therapeutic change requires hard, concerted and sustained effort. You encourage them to put up with personal discomfort and to engage in challenging but not overwhelming assignments.

You teach clients that while they may legitimately rate their deeds, acts and performances, they cannot helpfully rate their 'selves' because their 'self' is not a static entity but a changing process which executes millions of 'good' and 'bad' *acts* and which is too complex to be judged globally. Once clients internalize such a profound philosophic change, they accept themselves and others as fallible human beings, and habitually test the usefulness of their hypotheses about themselves, others and the world. By changing their dogmatic shoulds, oughts and musts to *preferences* they tend to minimally disturb themselves for the rest of their lives.

While this elegant solution may well be the most far-reaching way of achieving radical personality change, not all your clients are willing, or indeed able, to make such a radical shift in their personality. In such cases, you may realistically settle for helping some clients to change their interpretations about the stressors in their lives, and/or to modify their behaviour so that they get some immediate benefit from the therapeutic process. If you help your clients achieve a less elegant solution, they may remain vulnerable to future disturbance because they have not addressed their core musturbatory and dogmatic demands that they make about themselves, others and the world. You may, however, sensibly – and rationally! – compromise and not dogmatically insist that your clients always work towards addressing and overcoming their core musturbatory cognitions.

Wherever possible, however, try to encourage clients to internalize the Three Major Anti-Musturbatory Insights of REBT:

(a) Past or present activating negative events or stressors do not directly cause people's disturbances. No, it is their Belief System about these Adversities that largely unduly stresses them.

(b) Irrespective of how people disturbed themselves in the past, they *now* upset themselves largely because they *keep* reindoctrinating themselves with their Irrational Beliefs about past and present events.

(c) Because people are fallible humans, they very *easily* tend to *cling* to their self-defeating thoughts, feelings and actions. Nevertheless, they can work *hard and repeatedly* to dispute their Irrational Beliefs and can counteract their effects by strongly *acting* against them.

The importance of bibliotherapy and client homework assignments in counselling

Since REBT is a psychoeducational form of counselling in which clients actively participate in the learning process, you normally ask clients to read various REBT books and/or to listen to REBT lectures on audiotape. This may be done at any stage in the counselling process but is often done as part of the process of educating clients concerning the 'ABCs' of REBT. Such assignments can also be part of the other homework which clients are routinely encouraged to carry out in between counselling sessions. The material you select as bibliotherapy and the homework assignments themselves are to be carefully chosen for their relevance to your client's current problem and matched to his or her ability to readily understand them.

Recommended reading material and useful sources of information are preceded by an asterisk (*) in the References.

REBT counsellors attach a good deal of importance to encouraging clients to put into practice between sessions what they have learned within sessions. Ellis reported empirical data which suggested that clients who carry out homework assignments in cognitively oriented approaches to counselling gain more from counselling than clients who do not do homework.[12] Encouraging your clients to execute properly negotiated and well-designed homework assignments is an essential part of the counselling process.[13] Matters related to executing homework assignments will be discussed in greater detail at the appropriate stage in the following 13 steps of the counselling sequence.

THE 13 STEPS

We now focus on the 13 steps of the counselling sequence.[14] We recommend that from the outset you seek your client's agreement to tape record the sessions so that each of you has a record of what transpired during the sessions. This enables you (and your supervisor) to review progress and gives the client the opportunity to revise what he learned during the session and to pick up any points he may have missed or overlooked. Stress, of course, the issue of confidentiality and assure the client that taped material will not be used without his permission.

Table 3.1 below lists the 13 steps of the counselling sequence.

Table 3.1 *The rational emotive behaviour sequence*

Step 1: Ask for a problem
Step 2: Define and agree upon the target problem
Step 3: Assess C
Step 4: Assess A
Step 5: Identify and assess any secondary emotional problems
Step 6: Teach the B–C connection
Step 7: Assess Beliefs
Step 8: Connect Irrational Beliefs and C
Step 9: Dispute Irrational Beliefs
Step 10: Prepare your client to deepen conviction in Rational Beliefs
Step 11: Encourage your client to put new learning into practice
Step 12: Check homework assignments
Step 13: Facilitate the working through process

Step 1: Ask for a problem

Once you have welcomed your client, we suggest that you ask your client what problem she wants to talk about. Clients seldom come to counselling with just one problem. The problem she mentions may or may not be her most serious problem.

Asking your client what problem she would like to discuss first communicates three messages. First, your problem-focused stance conveys that you are both here to get a specific job done – that is, to help the client to overcome her emotional problem. Second, getting straight to the point illustrates that REBT is an efficient and focused approach to problem-solving and that you don't intend to waste time beating about the bush. Third, it sets the tone of what is to follow by indicating that you as the counsellor are taking an active part in directing your client to an immediate discussion of her problem.

Some clients may be reluctant to disclose a problem at first. In that case it may be helpful to ask what your clients hopes to achieve from counselling. If he reveals a goal you could then ask him to tell you in what ways he is not presently achieving his goal. You then may be able to identify feelings or behaviours that appear to be impeding the client from achieving his goal. If your client is hesitant about identifying a problem for discussion it may be helpful to ask him to fill in a Stress Map. Stress mapping was developed by Stephen Palmer[15] to aid assessment and problem definition. A completed example is shown in Box 3.1. (See also Appendix 7.)

The value of stress mapping is that it enables you to pinpoint various aspects of your client's life which seem to be prime sources of stress for him. Once he agrees with this preliminary identification of his stress trigger spots, you may then proceed to assess his ABCs in the usual way.

Step 2: Define and agree upon the target problem

Once you are given a problem or issue your client wants to talk about, arriving at a common understanding of the nature of the problem and an agreement to work on it builds a therapeutic alliance from the outset. Macaskill emphasizes the importance of educating clients about what to expect from rational emotive behaviour therapy (REBT).[16]

Since clients come to therapy with differing and sometimes distorted expectations about psychotherapy, you may decide at this point to educate your client about REBT. If your client's ideas on what counselling should be and what she wants to achieve from it significantly vary from the principles and practice of REBT, and if she is unwilling to open-mindedly give it a try, you may judiciously refer her to another counsellor.

However, if your client seems amenable to learning about REBT, you may begin to teach the ABCs at this stage, but be aware that your client may raise serious objections to its philosophy. For example, a client may state that she has a problem with performance anxiety. She admits to procrastinating over getting down to work on composing a musical score she had contracted to write, because she fears that by becoming more organized and efficient she would appear 'selfish' and would have to devote less time to meeting the demands of friends and family. She also feels that behaving efficiently would make her a 'robot' and destroy her musical creativity!

Take clients' reservations and fears seriously if you want to maintain the therapeutic alliance. Anticipate clients' misconceptions and difficulties, and be prepared to deal with them in an understanding and empathic manner.

Some clients may have certain practical problems as well as the psychological problem they want help with. Explain that your usual goal is to help them overcome psychological problems first and that, as you are accomplishing this, the client will

Box 3.1 *Stress mapping*

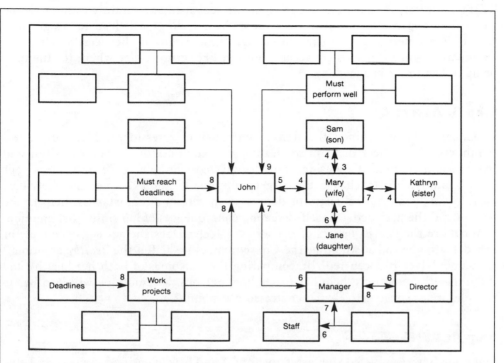

A stress map is a visual means of representing the sources of stress in your life. The central box represents yourself and the other boxes represent people you are in contact with. The other boxes can represent other potential stressors too, such as new computers or internal demands you place on yourself e.g. perfectionist beliefs.

Complete the boxes and then rate the amount of stress each other potential stressor can cause you on a scale of 1 to 10, where 10 represents high levels of stress. Place the score next to the appropriate stressor. Then ask youself how much stress you may cause the other people on your stress map. Also note these scores down.

Once the exercise is completed, note down any insights that you may have gained from undertaking stress mapping.

Source: Palmer, 1990

be in a healthier frame of mind with which to tackle her practical problems satisfactorily.

Once you and your client have identified and agreed upon a target problem, see that it is an unhealthy negative emotion and not a healthy reaction to some stressor. Take time to explain this difference and see that your client understands why unhealthy negative emotions are targeted for change. You may also work at changing unhealthy positive feelings, such as grandiosity and mania, although they are less common than the disturbed negative feelings. Help your client to understand that REBT definitely does *not* encourage clients to feel apathetic, unduly calm or serene when they experience negative life events. Such feelings will lead to resignation, rather than determination to try to change these events if they can be changed. Resignation will *not* help them accept, but not like, grim reality when, for the time being, it cannot be changed.

Step 3: Assess C

In Chapter 2 we outlined the REBT approach to assessment. Here are a few reminders. First, check that you are dealing with an unhealthy negative emotion and that you and your client are using similar language to describe it. Second, check your client's motivation to change the target emotion. If, for example, she feels it is 'healthy' or 'good' to feel angry or depressed in certain circumstances, help her to understand the destructive or self-defeating consequences of her unhealthy emotion.

What are the Consequences of the way she feels? Does she act constructively or self-defeatingly? What would be the Consequences if she felt the *healthy* emotion if the same Adversity occurred? By comparing the outcomes of both her healthy and the unhealthy emotions, help her to see how her healthy emotions will lead her to respond more constructively to her stressors at point A.

Step 4: Assess A

Once you have completed your assessment of A and have identified the part of A that triggered B, using the methods outlined in Chapter 2, try to reassess the client's goal for change. After you do inference chaining, the C which the client is most distressed about may well have changed. In that case, you now check with your client that his new goal is to change his disturbed C to a healthy response to the activating A.

As an example, let's look at how an REBT therapist would analyse the situation we described in Chapter 1 in which John needlessly stressed himself over the possibility of having to cancel his holiday. John has already described to the therapist what happened, so he takes it from there.

Therapist: When did you first begin to feel anxious about missing your flight?
John: Well, it wasn't when my aunt discovered she had forgotten her prescription for her heart pills. We had arrived at the airport early and it seemed to me at the time that we might be able to obtain an emergency supply. It was later, when I discovered that the stupid arrangements at the airport meant we would have to travel to another terminal to find a pharmacy, that I began to experience anxiety.
Therapist: Yes, you explained how you encountered certain difficulties in travelling with your aunt to this other terminal and locating the pharmacy where you hoped to obtain the necessary medication for your aunt. And at this point you said you also began to feel very angry. Also, your anxiety was mounting, right?
John: Yes.
Therapist: (probing for a possible link between the client's anger and his anxiety): You attributed the cause of your anger to your LFT. There *shouldn't be* so many

hassles to overcome, and you *should* be able to solve them quickly and easily with the minimum of inconvenience to yourself, is what I recall you said.

John: Yes.

Therapist: And as your anxiety increased, so did your anger, right?

John: Yes.

Therapist: Now, suppose that while you were in the middle of all those difficulties you mentioned, you suddenly heard an airport announcement that your flight had been delayed for at least six hours due to technical problems. Would you still have felt so anxious about missing your flight?

John: Well, no. With all that extra time at our disposal there would have been time to acquire my aunt's medication, or, failing that, there would have been time to notify her son of the problem. Perhaps he could have obtained the pills my aunt needed from his own physician and brought them to the airport.

Therapist: So your anxiety over missing your plane would have diminished. And how about your anger at what you called the 'stupid' arrangements implemented at the airport by the company controlling the pharmacies?

John: I would not have felt so angry then. I'd still have felt pretty pissed off with the planners responsible for such a cockeyed arrangement whereby passengers arriving at North Terminal have to make a special journey to South Terminal to obtain medicines on prescription and therby lose precious time as well as adding to the pressures on passengers already arriving at South Terminal with their own urgent prescriptions. But, no, I would not have felt so angry in the sense of wanting to wring the necks of these so-called planners as I actually did feel at the time.

Therapist: So your anger subsided with your anxiety. It seems that your anger at the world, or more specifically, at the faceless people responsible for providing emergency prescription facilities at the airport, although caused in the first instance by your Irrational Beliefs connected to your LFT, nevertheless was driven by your anxiety. For as your anxiety level dropped, so did your anger. Tell me, what was so anger- and anxiety-provoking about getting the medication too late to enable you to catch your plane, or even not getting the medication at all and still having to cancel your trip?

John: Because it would be a disaster for me! I'd lose my one and only chance in the year to have my holiday in Florida and I'd probably lose all the money I'd paid for my air fare, because I had no official status as a minder for my partially invalid aunt.

Therapist: That's why it would be annoying and unfortunate for you to lose your holiday through missing your flight. But why would it be a disaster?

John: Because I would feel such a fool! Think what my friends would say if I came home and told them that, despite arriving at the airport ahead of practically every other passenger booked on my flight, I still managed to miss my flight and screw up my entire holiday. They would think I must be some kind of prize idiot. And they would be right!

Therapist: Now we have the C: Feelings of self-pity, self-depreciation, low self-worth. You saw there was a possibility of losing your flight and therefore your holiday as a threat to your 'self-esteem'. Your anger served to protect you from having to face the implications of this possibility. In REBT we call it 'ego-defensive' anger. Had you been more self-accepting you would have been annoyed and disappointed at losing the flight through no fault of your own, but you would not have been angry. Moreover, when it began to look as if there was a real danger that you would run out of time, you would have felt concerned, rather than anxious about losing your plane. Moreover, your concern would have motivated you to consider other possibilities if the medication your aunt required had been unavailable at the airport. Perhaps you could have placed your aunt in the care of the airport emergency medical facilities while you telephoned her son to come and collect her and take her home, thus allowing you to continue the journey on your own. But in your anxiety-driven state, you would have been unlikely to think of constructive responses to your dilemma. Instead, your ego anxiety caused you to obsess about the 'awfulness' of losing your holiday. Then your 'self-esteem' would have taken a dive if you had actually lost your holiday because you would have irrationally blamed yourself, your whole being, for presumably making a mistake and missing the trip.

We can use this illustration to introduce the following important theoretical construct:

Two fundamental human disturbances

According to rational emotive behaviour theory humans can make absolute demands on self, other people and the world. But these three demands can actually be put under two major categories: *ego disturbance* and *discomfort disturbance*.[17]

In ego disturbance – that is, a person's self-damning for not achieving success and winning others' approval – the person's self-damnation or self-denigration involves the process of giving the 'self' a global negative rating (e.g., 'I'm a fool' or 'I'm no good') and thereby rating the 'self' as being bad or unworthy.

In discomfort disturbance, your clients make demands on others and on the world – demands that comfort and easy life conditions must exist all the time. When these demands are not met – as almost often they are not – then they make themselves emotionally disturbed.

The rational and healthy alternative to ego disturbance is unconditional self-acceptance (USA) – preferably a steadfast refusal to give oneself any kind of overall rating whatever. The rational and healthy alternative to discomfort disturbance is the client's training himself or herself to fully accept inevitable discomfort – not for its own sake, but to aid goal attainment and long-range happiness.

Ego and discomfort disturbance often coexist and significantly interact to cause severe psychological problems, particularly problems about problems. Thus you can assume that most clients have *both* LFT and self-damnation and try to help your clients discover and undo both kinds of disturbance.

Step 5: Identify and assess any secondary emotional problems

Examples of secondary problems are depression about being depressed, guilty about being angry, ashamed about being jealous, discomfort depression or LFT about self-downing and so on. In effect, your client's primary emotional problem becomes an activating event for an Irrational Belief which in turn results in a secondary emotional problem.

You may decide to deal with the secondary problem first if you think it is likely to significantly interfere with the client's ability to deal with his primary problem. If so, explain to your client why you first wish to deal with his secondary problem and agree that this will now become your main focus.

Assuming you have correctly assessed **A** and **C** and that your client now understands that it is **B** not **A** that largely determines his **C**, you can now go ahead and assess her Irrational Beliefs.

NOTES

1. Ellis, 1979b, 1994a, 1995a, 1996.
2. Dryden and Gordon, 1990b.
3. Ellis, 1977c, 1982.
4. Ellis, 1972c.
5. Ellis, 1977c, p. 15.
6. Ellis, 1976, 1994a, 1996.
7. Ellis, 1995a, p. 12.
8. Ellis, 1985a, 1988, 1991b.
9. Ellis, 1990a, p. 81.
10. Dryden and Gordon, 1993b.
11. Dryden, 1987.
12. Ellis, 1983.
13. Dryden, 1990b.
14. Dryden, 1990b.
15. Palmer, 1990.
16. Macaskill, 1989.
17. Ellis, 1979b, 1980.

CHAPTER 4

The Middle Stage of Stress Counselling

There is no hard-and-fast dividing line separating the beginning stage of counselling from the middle stage. But after a few sessions of following the procedure just described, you are probably ready to move on. In the middle stage you will follow through on the client's target problem, engage the client in relevant tasks and begin work on her other problems.

Step 6: Teach the B–C connection

This step involves your teaching your client that his emotional problem is largely determined by his Beliefs rather than by the activating event that you have already assessed. To help people new to the practice of REBT there are several standard REBT texts to help teach the B–C connection, such as those by Dryden, Ellis, and Walen, DiGiuseppe and Dryden.[1] One commonly used teaching dialogue is The Money Example. Here it is in full.

THE MONEY EXAMPLE

Therapist: I would like to teach you a model which explains the main factors that account for people's emotional problems. Would you be interested in learning about it now?

Client: Yes.

Therapist: All right. Now there are four parts to this model. Here's part one. Imagine that you have £10 in your pocket and that you have the following belief: 'I prefer to have a minimum of £11 in my pocket, but it's not essential that I do so. It would be bad if I had less than my preferred £11 but it would hardly be the end of the world.' Now, if you really believed this, how would you feel about only having £10 when you prefer, but do not demand, that you must have a minimum of £11?

Client: I'd feel concerned if I only had £10.

Therapist: Right. Or you'd feel annoyed or disappointed, but you wouldn't kill yourself.

Client: Certainly not.

Therapist: OK. Now, let's take part two of the model. This time you hold a different belief.

This time you believe: 'I *absolutely must* have a minimum of £11 in my pocket at all times. I must! I must! I must! And it would be the end of the world if I had less.' Holding this belief, you look in your pocket and again find that you have only £10. Now, how would you feel this time about having £10 when you absolutely insisted that you must have £11?

Client: Very anxious.

Therapist: Right – or depressed. Now look carefully and observe something really important. Faced with the same situation (you have only £10 in your pocket) different beliefs lead to different feelings. Now, here is part three of the model. This time you still have exactly the same belief as you did a moment ago in part two of the model, namely: 'I *absolutely must* have a minimum of £11 in my pocket at all times. I must! I must! I must! And it would be the end of the world if I had less.' This time, however, in checking the contents of your pocket you find you've got £12. Two one-pound coins are lying under your £10 note. How would you feel now about having £12 when you absolutely insist on having a minimum of £11 in your pocket at all times?

Client: Relieved, content.

Therapist: Right. Now, here is the fourth and final part of the model. With that same £12 in your pocket and that same belief, namely: 'I absolutely must have a minimum of £11 in my pocket at all times. I must! I must! I must! And it would be the end of the world if I had less', something would occur to you that would lead you to be very anxious again. What do you think that might be?

Client: Oh, let me see now. I believe I must have a minimum of £11 on me at all times. I've got more than the minimum, yet I'm getting very anxious again. Oh! I get it. What if I lose £2? I'm scared I might lose £2. Is that it?

Therapist: Right. Or you might spend £2 or you might get robbed or mugged. Now the point of this model is this. Practically all humans, black or white, rich or poor, male or female make themselves disturbed when they don't get what they believe they must get. They are also vulnerable to making themselves disturbed when they do have what they believe they must have, because they could always lose it.

Client: I see. So, this means that not only will I be unhappy by making myself disturbed when I don't get what I believe I must have, but even when I do get what I believe I must have, I'm likely to become or remain anxious because I can always lose it.

Therapist: Right. If humans would stick rigorously (but not rigidly) to their non-demanding preferences and not transmute them into musts, they will feel healthily concerned when they don't get what they prefer and will be able to take constructive action to change these conditions or to prevent undesirable consequences in future. Is that clear?

Client: Yes.

Therapist: Well, in case I haven't made my point clearly enough can you explain it back to me in your own words?

There are several important points to be noted here. First, this dialogue has been carefully constructed to teach clients the ABCs of REBT as succinctly and as clearly as possible. Since accurate assessment of the client's problems is so important, you'd better develop the ability to clearly teach clients the ABCs of REBT. Use the Money Example or some other effective analogy to do so. As Dryden observes:

The money example, when presented correctly, is a potent way of teaching the ABC model. However, it is difficult to master and trainees do have difficulty in learning it. When they practise it they tend to make a number of errors.[2]

Here are some errors that Dryden examines.

COMMON ERRORS IN TEACHING THE MONEY EXAMPLE

1. *Failure to distinguish fully between Rational and Irrational Beliefs.*   When asked to explain the Money Example in their own words, a common mistake made by clients is to describe only the first part of the Rational Belief which asserts the person's preference, namely: 'I would prefer to have a minimum of £11 on me at all times.' REBT theory states that people can easily change their preferences to demands. A major way of guarding against this when teaching the Money Example is to take care to negate the person's demand as well as asserting his preference. For example, you can say 'I would prefer to have a minimum of £11 on me at all times, but it is not essential that I do so'. Those last nine words meet the requirement for completeness of the primary part of the Rational Belief or preference.

According to REBT theory, preferences are primary Rational Beliefs, which have several rational derivatives, especially anti-awfulizing, high frustration tolerance and unconditional self-acceptance (USA) and unconditional other acceptance (UOA). To reinforce her understanding of the full Rational Belief, encourage your client to state the anti-awfulizing derivative: 'It would be bad to have less than my preferred £11, but it would not be the end of the world.' Putting several rational self-statements together, your client can arrive at the full expression of her Rational Belief: 'I would prefer to have a minimum of £11 on me at all times, but it is not essential that I do so. It would be unfortunate to have less than my preferred £11 but it would not be the end of the world.'

2. *Failure to clarify vague descriptions of emotions.*   When clients fail to clarify their emotions they will be unable to clearly distinguish healthy from unhealthy negative emotions. For example, you might ask your client to imagine he has £10 in his pocket and to have this Belief: 'I would prefer to have a minimum of £11 on me at all times, but it is not essential that I do so. It would be bad to have less than my preferred £11, but it would not be the end of the world.' You then put the question: 'Now if you really believed this, how would you feel about only having £10 when you want, but do not demand, a minimum of £11?' The client may answer 'Upset'.

When your client uses the word 'upset' you have no means of knowing whether this refers to a healthy negative feeling like concern, disappointment and annoyance, or to an unhealthy negative feeling like anxiety, anger or feelings of self-pity. If you allow the client to use the vague word 'upset' you will find it difficult to show her that Irrational Beliefs lead primarily to disturbed emotions.

To avoid confusion, clarify what your client means by 'upset' and encourage her to use more precise terms such as concerned or anxious, annoyed or angry and so on. By doing so you help your client to distinguish healthy from unhealthy emotions and pave the way to her seeing the connection between these two kinds of emotion and the Rational and Irrational Beliefs that accompany them.

3. *Failure to emphasize the irrational components of clients' Beliefs.* Just as clients will sometimes fail to fully articulate their Rational Beliefs or preferences, so too may they fail to express their Irrational Beliefs. When your client is invited to feed back to you his understanding of the ABC model in his own words, his must is often weakly or insipidly expressed. Because of this insufficient emphasis, repetition is used in the model – I must! I must! I must! Expressions such as 'absolutely must' also bring out the essentially dogmatic, commanding essence of the word. Encourage your client to emphasize the awfulizing derivative of his must – 'and it would be the end of the world'. Stating this helps to emphasize the irrationality of musturbation.

Step 7: Assess Beliefs

Let us remind you of the material covered in Chapter 2:

1. Help your client to distinguish clearly between her Rational and Irrational Beliefs. Encourage her to explain in her own words the difference between the two kinds of Belief. As an exercise, ask her to write down the distinguishing features of rationality and irrationality.
2. See that she understands both the core philosophy of Irrational Beliefs – that is, her dogmatic musts, absolute shoulds, and oughts – and the four main derivatives from these basic premises: awfulizing, I-can't-stand-it-itis, damnation of self, others and the world, and always and never thinking.
3. Check that you and the client are both using words carrying the same meaning. You can either persuade her to use the REBT terminology of emotions, or you may choose to adopt her terms for describing her feelings. Whatever route you take, be consistent in your usage and be careful to ensure that unhealthy negative emotions are accurately identified and referred to by using agreed-upon words.
4. Remind your client that not all uses of the words 'must', 'should' and 'ought' are necessarily linked to Irrational Beliefs and that these words have several different meanings in the English language. Rational emotive behaviour theory states that only *absolute* shoulds and musts lead to emotional disturbance.

     You can give your client examples of the legitimate use of 'should' when the word is used (a) to indicate a preference ('I should take this road rather than that one'). (b) When it is used in an empirical sense to indicate a law of nature ('When uranium-235 reaches its critical mass a nuclear explosion should occur'). (c) When it is used as a recommendation ('You should see the play that is showing at our local theatre').
5. Remember the Three Basic Musts leading to core Irrational Beliefs. Point out that virtually all IBs are variants of these Three Major Irrational Beliefs. That should help your client to more easily identify her and other people's irrational beliefs.

ASSESSING IBS BY USING QUESTIONS

As noted in Chapter 2 the advantage of using open-ended questions to assess your client's IBs is that you are unlikely to put words into your client's mouth about his belief. The disadvantage is that your client is likely to respond to your question with another inference about his **A** rather than articulate a strongly held Irrational Belief.

'What were you telling yourself to make yourself anxious at **A**?' The answer might be 'Trying to get emergency medication in this place is such a blasted time-wasting nuisance that I could miss my flight!' This answer is part observation and inference, and does not fully articulate an Irrational Belief. You may then explain to your client that his answer is not an IB and briefly explain to him how to look for his Irrational Belief about **A**.

You may prefer to ask theory-driven questions to arrive at the client's IB. 'What *demand* were you making about the situation you were in to make yourself disturbed?' This may unearth more than one demand: 'I've just got to get on that plane!' 'It *shouldn't be* so damned difficult and time-consuming to obtain the medication my aunt needs!' If you focus on disputing one demand at a time, including the destructive conclusions based on it, you will arrive at the core Irrational Belief(s).

The danger of using theory-driven questions is that you may be putting words into your client's mouth and attributing to her Irrational Beliefs that she may not actually have. However, if it is clear from your assessment that your client does have an unhealthy negative emotion at **C** this danger will be minimized. A useful theory-driven question to assess the presence to a derivative from a must is: 'What kind of person did you think you would be if you did miss your flight?'

Step 8: Connect IB and C

Here your aim is to help your client to understand the connection between his Irrational Beliefs and his disturbed emotions at **C**. Once your client understands that so long as he makes demands upon himself, others or the world, he will probably make himself disturbed; and once he sees that if he wants to minimize his disturbances he can change his Beliefs, you can proceed to the next stage where you begin to show him how to dispute his Irrational Beliefs.

At this stage, your client will probably only lightly be convinced of her Rational Beliefs. That is, it makes sense 'intellectually', but not 'emotionally'. Encourage your client to see that even her light conviction is a sign of progress, but that when she makes her conviction deeper and stronger – as she tends to do with work and persistent practice at disputing and acting against her Irrational Beliefs – real emotional and behavioural change is likely to follow.

When dealing with your client's target problem help her to understand, or remind her of, the main refutation of Irrational Beliefs:

There is no evidence in support of absolutist demands nor of the self-sabotaging conclusions derived from them.

Step 9: Dispute Irrational Beliefs

As you proceed to show your client how to vigorously Dispute his IBs, we once more remind you of the distinction between changing perceptions of Adversities (**As**) and changing Beliefs (**Bs** about these perceptions). This distinction encourages elegant rather than inelegant solutions to **Cs**. Once you help your client to restruc ture his core **Bs** – which is your primary task – you may help him also see his **As** differently. For example, once your client is convinced that there is nothing *terrible* or *awful* about making mistakes, you may help him to see that his 'great errors' were minor or that he can advantageously learn from them.

TACKLE ONE IB AT A TIME

As you show your client how to dispute his IBs, usually concentrate on one at a time. Dispute this IB fully and check that your client reduces it before you switch to another IB. If you switch from one IB to another before you have really finished with the first your client will often be confused.

USE THREE DISPUTING STRATEGIES

Once again, show your client the three main forms of Disputing: (1) *logical* – because she *wants* something 'good' to happen, it doesn't *have* to occur; (2) *empirical* – nothing that she wants actually *must* exist; (3) *pragmatic* – if she holds absolute *musts* and concludes that it's *terrible* when they are not fulfilled she will make herself miserable and less effective. Useful questions you can ask your clients, or encourage them to ask themselves, are:

Empirical
- Where is the evidence that you must ...?
- Is there a law of the universe that states that you must ...?
- Where is the evidence that you can't stand it?
- How long have you been standing it?
- I can understand why it's bad, but how does that make it awful?

Logical
- Where is the logic that you should?
- Just because something is bad, does it logically follow that it's really the end of the world or awful?
- Is it good logic to believe that because you want ... therefore you must ...?

Pragmatic
- Where will it get you if you hold the belief that I must ... that I can't stand it ... that it's awful ... that I'm worthless?
- How is believing that you must ... going to help you achieve your long-term/ healthy goals?
- What's in it for you, if you give up this idea?

DEVELOP RATIONAL ALTERNATIVE BELIEFS

Once your client has successfully disputed an Irrational Belief he had better replace it with a Rational Belief. Otherwise, his old Irrational Belief will probably return to plague him. When your client has made some progress in replacing an Irrational Belief with a new Rational Belief, encourage him to dispute *it* logically, empirically and pragmatically. Doing this will help him see for himself that his new Rational Beliefs are in fact self-helping and can stand up to examination, whereas his Irrational Beliefs cannot.

The bottom line in disputing is to help your client clearly recognize and acknowledge that her 'stressed' condition does not merely stem from *disliking* the stressors in her life and strongly *desiring* to remove or modify them. More importantly, they stem from her demanding, insisting and commanding that such stressors should, ought and must not exist, and from 'catastrophizing' about the 'horror' and 'awfulness' of their actuality as Ellis points out.[3]

To give you an idea of what we mean by showing the client how to dispute his Irrational Beliefs, we will focus on the example we described in Chapter 1 and continued in Chapter 3. John is the client in the dialogue that follows.

AN EXAMPLE OF DISPUTING

Therapist: OK, John, You've told me that you arrived at the airport in plenty of time because you believe in allowing for the usual unforeseeable delays and hassles that can occur on a journey to an international airport. Taking sensible precautions to arrive in good time for an important journey indicates a sensible degree of concern. However, your concern soon changed to anxiety when something happened to interrupt your plans.

John: Yes. I felt shocked when my aunt discovered that she had forgotten her heart pills and that she could not continue her journey without them. But my feelings of anxiety did not begin immediately but soon afterwards, when I discovered how difficult and time-consuming it was going to be to obtain an emergency supply of her medication. Then, as time went on and we seemed no nearer to a solution to the problem, I became very angry.

Therapist: OK. Which emotional problem would you like to deal with first?

John: I would like to deal with the anger first. I don't like feeling angry. I get a destructive feeling in my gut.

Therapist: All right. What was it about the stress that you described that triggered your anger? The situation contributed to, but did not *make* you angry. What were you telling yourself as you hustled your semi-invalid aunt around the airport terminals while you sought emergency medication for her?

John: I kept thinking 'This is a right pain in the behind. Why does getting a simple prescription have to be so bloody difficult?'

Therapist: All right, we accept that getting your aunt an emergency prescription for her heart pills was difficult. But how were you making yourself angry about it?

John: Because this situation didn't just happen. It was planned. The company that runs the pharmacy in the South Terminal also runs the pharmacy in the North Terminal, so it makes no sense to authorize only one outlet to fill passengers' prescriptions. Such an arrangement practically ensures delays for any passengers whose flights leave from North Terminal, as well as delaying passengers whose flights leave from South Terminal, because *all* passengers are forced to line up in one queue at the only outlet dispensing prescription medicines.

Therapist: Yes, but you haven't answered my question. You've explained why you, and probably most people, would be frustrated by these difficulties and why it *would be better* if they did not exist. My question to you was, what was it about that admittedly difficult situation that triggered (but did not cause) your anger?

John: *It shouldn't have been* so difficult! Surely anyone with an ounce of planning sense could have foreseen that the arrangement they came up with would create all kinds of unnecessary problems! I think it's *awful* that my aunt's health should be put in jeopardy – to say nothing of the loss of my flight, my only chance of a holiday this year, and the loss of my air fare money. *I can't stand* being put in this situation through no fault of my own, and the people responsible for this idiotic piece of so-called planning *ought to* be slung out on their ears!

Therapist: Well, with these demands you are practically certain to make yourself angry. You told me that you don't like feeling angry because it creates a destructive feeling in your gut. So would you like me to show you how you can stop yourself feeling angry the next time your wishes are frustrated?

John: Yes, I've always found it easy to become angry when other people act in what I consider a stupid or inefficient manner. That causes me quite a problem!

Therapist: Well, there are several issues here. I noticed that in damning the people who you assumed were responsible for planning the facilities for obtaining emergency medication, you made a number of inferences or assumptions. For example, you inferred that the difficulties you and your aunt encountered were due to bad planning. That is possible, but there could be other explanations. For example, there might be a temporary shortage of trained staff which led to only one pharmacy being available to deal with emergency medical prescriptions.

John: I never thought of that.

Therapist: No. You see, when people hold Irrational Beliefs, these Beliefs tend to lead to distorted assumptions about the Activating Events. They attribute motives and intentions to others which may not in fact exist. Before making accusations, it is a good idea to check your facts. And be careful with your assumptions and inferences!

John: Yes, I see that. There could have been other reasons for the difficulties we experienced.

Therapist: Right. But let's get back to what you were telling yourself to make yourself angry about your difficult experiences. First, let's assume that the planners got it wrong and that the difficulties you and your aunt experienced were entirely due to bad planning, bad management, or both.

John: Right, I'll go along with that.

Therapist: Now, why *shouldn't* these difficulties and hassles you described exist?

John: Uh, well, because without these hassles, there would be less delay in obtaining emergency medicines and less risk of people missing their flights. Obtaining emergency medication from, say, two sensibly located pharmacies, would be easier for everybody. With things as they are now, you could easily lose time and money and even your flight through no fault of your own.

Therapist: Yes, but you are only telling me that one set of planning arrangements would get good results, while another set would get poor results. You still haven't told me why a good time-saving plan *absolutely must* exist.

John: Well, yes, I think I see what you're saying. If hassles exist, then delays are inevitable.

Therapist: But underneath I can still hear you saying 'But unnecessary hassles *shouldn't* exist!'

John: You're right, they damned well *shouldn't*!

Therapist: But your Belief that hassles and difficulties shouldn't exist, makes no sense. Can you see why?

John: Not really.

Therapist: Well, let's look closely at what you're telling yourself. You obviously wish that these hassles didn't exist. They caused you and your aunt considerable inconvenience. Now, does it logically follow that because you strongly wish that certain difficulties did not exist, therefore they *absolutely must* not exist?

John: No, I guess not. If I want something it does not logically follow that I absolutely must get it.

Therapist: Right. Now look at your Belief from another point of view. 'These hassles *shouldn't* exist' – was what you said. Hassles exist, don't they?

John: No doubt about it!

Therapist: Right. What exists, exists. Therefore it makes no sense to say something shouldn't exist when it definitely does exist.

John: I can see, now that you point it out, that hassles really should exist, if they do. No matter how much I don't *like* them to or *wish* they didn't exist.

Therapist: That's right. You can legitimately wish or prefer that certain hassles didn't exist, but when you insist that they *absolutely shouldn't* exist, you are setting up a law to that effect. Obviously, there is no such law, for if there were, then hassles could not possibly exist. Since they undoubtedly do exist, there is no law – except the law you set up in your head! Do you run the universe?

John: OK, I accept your point and I can see that my belief that hassles shouldn't exist is irrational and cannot be supported. My goal is to get rid of my anger. So if I give up my demanding that hassles like I described should not exist, will that help?

Therapist: Yes, but more than that is required. There's your *awfulizing* about the possible loss of your holiday. Is it really 'awful' – meaning *totally* bad or badder than it should be if you missed your flight and had to forgo your holiday for another year? That's what 'awful' really means: as bad as it *could* be, worse than it *absolutely should* be.

John: No, it's not awful. It's bad but not 100 per cent bad, I have to admit.

Therapist: Right. Nothing can be badder than it actually is, badder than it *should* be. Even 100 per cent bad would be almost impossible to reach. If you missed your flight, lost your holiday and your money, many worse things could happen to you. For example, in hurrying to catch your plane, you could slip and break your leg! Or your aunt might have a cardiac arrest and have to be rushed to hospital. No matter what misfortunes befall you, things could always be worse.

John: Most people would say that death was 100 per cent bad, but I can see that some people might even welcome it – like terminally ill people suffering great pain from an inoperable cancer, for example.

Therapist: Quite so. And can you see that your Belief that you *can't stand* having your holiday disrupted through no fault of your own, is utter nonsense? If you think about it, you *can* stand anything that happens to you until you die. And *'I can't stand it!'* means that I couldn't be happy at all if I had to postpone my trip. Is *that* true?

John: No. I see what you mean. I'm really acting crazy when I say 'I *can't stand* real frustration!' when I actually am standing it!

Therapist: OK. Now what about your damning comments about the people who allegedly screwed up on the planning of passenger access to emergency prescription medication?

John: Well, I think it could have been handled better.

Therapist: Perhaps. But even assuming that some people did a bad job of planning these access arrangements, how does that make them *damnable people*? Are they *total no-goodniks*?

John: You mean, even if they made a big mistake?

Therapist: I mean regardless of whether they made a big mistake, or a little mistake. The size of the mistake is irrelevant. If they made *any* kind of mistake, including a big one, why does that make them worthless individuals, deserving of nothing but censure and damnation?

John: Well, when I think about it, I suppose nobody is really worthless because they make mistakes.

Therapist: Why?

John: I imagine it's because we do millions of things, some good, some bad, throughout our life and it wouldn't be right to judge people as basically good or bad merely on the basis of just some of the things they do, or the traits they possess.

Therapist: You're almost there. You cannot legitimately judge people at all by giving them some kind of global rating. Humans are very complex and keep changing all the time. You can judge or rate a person's traits, deeds and abilities according to some standard. For example, you can rate a tennis player's ability or a musician's technique and so on, but you cannot rate a person's totality.

John: I see. So that means that if someone acts foolishly, for example, their foolish act in no way makes them a *fool*?

Therapist: Correct. It is a gross overgeneralization to equate a person's totality or personhood with some of his performances or attributes. You can rate a person's *deeds*, but not the *person* who performs those deeds. We are all fallible human beings. If you can learn to accept yourself and others as fallible, mistake-making humans – for that is our nature – you will become less prone to condemn yourself or others when they act stupidly or inefficiently. And you will become less prone to whine about the hassles you encounter when life conditions are not as fair or as comfortable and easy as you would wish them to be.

John: OK, I'll try to remember that. Could we discuss my anxiety now, seeing that was a problem for me at the time?

Therapist: Yes, but there are two more things I suggest we do before that. You have seen how your anger stemmed from your Irrational Beliefs – your dictates that the hassles and difficulties you encountered at the airport *absolutely must not* exist. Intellectually – or lightly – you may now see that those IBs simply don't make sense. But it will take time, and considerable work and practice at disputing your IBs, before a more rational set of beliefs begins to 'sink in' to your head and heart. I'm going to give you an exercise now to help that process on its

	way. Then I suggest you come up with a rational alternative set of Beliefs to your previous IBs that caused your anger. Does that make sense?
John:	Yes. I'd better finish dealing with my anger before we go on to tackle my anxiety.
Therapist:	All right. This exercise is called Rational Emotive Imagery, or REI for short. This is what you do. Close your eyes and imagine youself back in the situation at the airport. Imagine that things are even worse than they were and everything is blocking you from getting your aunt's medication. Can you vividly imagine that happening?
John:	Yes, I see it very clearly.
Therapist:	Fine, how do you honestly *feel* as you imagine you and your aunt being needlessly blocked and about to miss your plane?
John:	Very angry. In fact enraged!
Therapist:	Good! Feel as enraged as you can. Really feel it, feel it!
John:	Oh, I really do!
Therapist:	Fine. Now keep the same very frustrating image in mind – don't change it! – and make yourself feel *only* annoyed and disappointed about what is happening. Not angry, *only* healthily annoyed and disappointed.
John:	I'm having great difficulty giving up my anger. At this rate, we're going to miss our flight, and my holiday with it, damn them!
Therapist:	Yes, but you can always control your feelings. It's not what happens to you, but how you *feel* about it. So I want you to change your feeling of anger only to annoyance and disappointment. It may be difficult, but you can do it. Keep working at it until you feel annoyed and displeased, but not angry. *Just* very annoyed and disappointed but not enraged. You can do it! Tell me when you feel only annoyed and disappointed, but not angry.
John:	(signalling with his hand): I've done that.
Therapist:	Now open your eyes and tell me what you did to change your angry feelings to feelings only of annoyance and disappointment.
John:	I was telling myself 'I wish this wasn't happening to me. We could do without all these delays and difficulties right now, but I suppose they are doing their best under difficult circumstances, so we'll just have to wait as patiently as we can. This is the way things are. If we miss our flight, that is just too bad, it's a real pain in the butt, but it isn't the end of the world. I guess we can stand the disappointment and later on maybe we can try to make the trip without these damned hassles.'
Therapist:	Good! Rational emotive imagery only takes a minute or two to do. So repeat it every day for 20 or 30 days – until you train yourself to feel automatically healthily annoyed, disappointed, displeased and regretful – instead of enraged and panicked – whenever you imagine a very frustrating event or you actually experience one.

REI can be used in conjunction with cognitive disputing to help your clients overcome many of their potential or actual disturbances about their stress-related problems, such as anxiety, worries about their health, and anger at life conditions. Clients benefit most from the *steady* practice of REI. A now-and-then use of REI will not be nearly as effective as regular, steady practice, preferably on a daily basis. By the steady use of

REI, clients can philosophically and emotionally acclimate themselves to virtually any kind of emotional disturbance that they are likely to help create.

Here are some more ways that you can help John with his problems:

Therapist: Now give some thought to what we were doing when we disputed your Irrational Beliefs that caused you to feel angry. Go over these disputes several times. You could tape record the Irrational Beliefs and then your disputes of these IBs. Then listen to your answers. How *forceful* and *convincing* are they? Did you miss anything out? If so, go back to basics and dispute your musts and their derivatives using the three strategies you've been learning (that is, the logical, the pragmatic and the consistent-with-reality strategies). And practise your REI every day until you really *see* and *feel* that the difficulties you experienced were just that – hassles that you *can* stand and cope with – instead of some kind of horror or utter catastrophe that you invented.

John: (some time later): I've been working on those exercises you suggested. I've also worked out a set of rational alternative Beliefs to my previous irrational ones, the IBs that created my anger. My new Rational Beliefs are: 'I would definitely prefer that the arrangements for passengers to obtain emergency medication at airports be situated at conveniently accessible pharmacies within the airport, but they don't *have to be*. If I am delayed by circumstances beyond my control and as a result I miss my flight and lose my vacation, that would be decidedly unfortunate, but it would not be *awful*, or *terrible*. I can obviously *stand*, though I shall never like, the loss of my vacation and any loss of money I would incur should I miss my flight. If it happens, it happens. Tough! I can still be happy in spite of this disappointment, and if it turns out that somebody in authority goofed over the locations of the pharmacies, he or she is not a damnable or worthless person, merely a quite fallible human being like the rest of us.'

Therapist: Now, that sounds like a more rational attitude. How would you now *feel* if you really keep that rational attitude?

John: Oh, definitely annoyed and very disappointed. As you know, I attached a lot of importance to going to the States at that time. It was the only time I could make the trip.

Therapist: As a result of your healthier feeling of annoyance and disappointment what *action* might you now consider taking to improve the situation at the airport, and possibly to reduce the risk of future disappointments?

John: Well, I could write to the pharmacy company responsible for making the arrangements for obtaining emergency medication at the airport. I could describe the facts, explain what happened to me and my aunt, point out the hassles for passengers of the company's current arrangements, and explain how I very nearly came to lose my flight because of these poor arrangements. And I could ask the pharmacy what actions they will take to avoid such difficulties arising in future.

Therapist: That sounds like a constructive attempt to improve the situation. You would not be angrily condemning the company or a particular individual for what happened, but merely describing the facts and asking them what they propose to do about improving the situation in future. With that more rational attitude, you would be more likely to elicit a constructive response from the management of the company than if you had hectored them over their 'horrible failures' and 'terrible inadequacies'.

To sum up, Disputing in REBT asks questions about clients' Irrational Beliefs, and doesn't merely replace them with rational alternatives. Your aim is mainly to teach your clients the art of scientific thinking, of devising hypotheses, and of looking for evidence for and against their hypotheses. The more skilled your clients become in this art of asking questions and falsifying their disturbance-creating assumptions, the better they will be at generalizing beyond their immediate Adversities to any later unfortunate Activating Experiences they may experience.

DISPUTING JOHN'S ANXIETY-CREATING BELIEFS

Here are some ways to reduce John's anxiety.

Therapist: You mentioned that you were anxious when the difficulties you encountered at the airport almost made you miss your flight. Is that correct?

John: Yes. Am I right in thinking that I could attack the relevant Irrational Beliefs that created my anxiety in the same way that you showed me how to reduce my anger?

Therapist: Yes. Can you now see that you were not merely wanting to catch your plane. You were *demanding* that you *must* do so.

John: Yes, and my demand for certainty probably added 'fuel to the fire', so to speak, when I was getting very angry at all those delays and hassles I was undergoing with my aunt.

Therapist: Exactly! Your 'stress', the anxiety that you created for yourself, arose not from your *desire* to make it to the plane on time but mainly from your *demanding*, your *insisting* that your arrangements proceed as planned, and that it would be *awful* if they didn't. Your anxiety, in the face of those 'stressful' conditions you encountered at the airport, arose mainly from your *need*, your *insistence* that you catch your plane on time and enjoy your planned vacation.

John: I see. And did my damning of the people I assumed were responsible for those hassle-filled arrangements at the airport arise from the same kind of certainty-demanding, absolutistic thinking I was indulging in at the time?

Therapist: Most probably. Your thoughts were 'I must, *absolutely must* catch my plane'. That was your core IB. Your derivatives consisted of self-defeating conclusions, such as 'It would be *awful* if I lost my holiday through missing my plane through no fault of mine! I *couldn't stand* that horror! I would feel such a fool if it happened!' Then you went back to 'So at all costs I *absolutely must* catch my plane!'

John: Yes, I seem to recall that's exactly what I was telling myself at the time I was feeling really anxious and stressed out. But what about my feeling that I'd look like and be a complete fool if I did miss the plane? How would I overcome that?

Therapist: You would apply the same rational reasoning as you did when you challenged the legitimacy of damning people on the grounds of their alleged stupidity. Let's just suppose that you missed your flight on account of some foolish act on your part. In fact, you don't seem to have acted all that foolishly. You were more the victim of circumstances, although some of your reactions were admittedly less than helpful because of your musts about the situation you found yourself in. But let's suppose you had acted foolishly. The relevant question to ask is, How can a foolish *act* make you a *fool*? A fool is, almost by definition, one who can *only* and *always* act foolishly – someone who has an *essence* of foolishness. You well may have done a number of foolish things. But we are all fallible humans. So how does one stupid act, or even several, make you a complete and utter *fool*?

John: It really doesn't is the answer, I suppose.

Therapist: Because?

John: Because labelling myself as *a fool* is a form of self-rating, which you have been teaching me is philosophically illegitimate. I'm really beginning to see now that I can legitimately rate my acts, deeds and performances, but not my 'self', my *totality*. Besides, as you've previously explained, it is a gross overgeneraliza- tion to take just one aspect of me – my foolish behaviour, and conclude that that is *equal* to my entire being. I am a complex entity, as all humans are, and my totality cannot be measured by or equated to any aspects of me – such as my thoughts, feelings, deeds, traits or performances.

Therapist: Right. I think you're beginning to get it now. Moreover, once you convince your- self that a foolish act cannot make you a *foolish person*, but merely a *person* who acts foolishly from time to time, you can accept yourself as an imperfect human being who occasionally behaves stupidly or ineptly but in no way is less worthy for doing so. Indeed, you can go a step further and drop the word 'worthy' altogether, as well as its opposite 'unworthy', and simply accept your- self without any ifs or buts whatever. You can say 'I exist. That is an empirically provable fact. And since I choose to continue to exist I can direct my life so that I minimize my pain and maximize my short- and long-range pleasures. In other words, I *choose* to remain alive and to enjoy myself. Now let me work out how I can most effectively use my REBT training to achieve these goals.'

John: Yes, without rating my *self*, my *me-ness*, or my *essence*, I'd like to really get hold of that philosophy. It makes a lot of sense to value my traits, deeds, acts and performances that enhance the quality of my life and to disvalue those behaviours that lessen my enjoyments and that bring me needless trouble and pain. Rating my acts and traits makes sense, while rating my 'self' doesn't. 'Life is short enough, so let's make it a real ball!' sounds like a great philosophy. But isn't this refusal to evaluate one's *self* difficult to achieve?

Therapist: In most instances, yes. In REBT we note that we humans rarely stop at rating our traits and deeds, but that we assume that we have a 'self' or 'ego' and that we have to rate *that*, too. so you'll have difficulty in becoming a person who *doesn't* rate yourself. But you can accomplish this difficult feat if you work and practise at it. I've already shown you how. It's now up to you to persistently work and practise at changing your self-defeating Irrational Beliefs and replac- ing them with more useful philosophies.

Let me hear what rational alternative Beliefs you have come up with now that you see that your anxiety is self-handicapping as well as giving you a needless pain in the gut.

John: OK. I'll go back to the beginning. Since I really wanted that holiday in the States I felt healthily concerned about the possibility of losing it. That is why I made special efforts to arrive with my aunt at the departure airport with plenty of time to spare. These days it makes sense to allow for transport delays and other hassles when you set out on an important journey. So I was somewhat concerned about encountering possible delays, but also determined to take all practicable steps to avoid them.

Therapist: OK. Now, what did you tell yourself to transmute that eminently sensible feeling of concern to one of gut-wrenching anxiety?

John: Well, as I said before, once I realized that we were up against real problems, and it began to look doubtful that we would even make it to the plane on time, I was saying to myself 'I *must*, I *absolutely must*, catch that plane and if I don't, that would be terrible!' I can *now* see why that belief is totally irrational. So, since I want to give up my musts and awfulizing and adopt a healthier and more constructive attitude of concern, I could choose to believe something like this: 'I strongly *prefer* to have my trip to the States work out as I've planned, but it *doesn't have to*. If circumstances outside my control result in my losing my holiday, it is certainly unfortunate because of the loss of time and money I shall incur, but it isn't a disaster. I won't like forgoing my trip for another year but I can obviously stand the disappointment. Perhaps I could have acted more effectively had I not been consumed by anxiety and later, by anger, over the poor arrangements for obtaining emergency medication, but I am not a *fool* for behaving stupidly or ineffectively. I accept myself as a fallible person with my poor performance on this occasion but in no way will I denigrate myself for it.'

Therapist: That's better. With that more rational attitude, how might you have acted more constructively to achieve a better outcome, given your circumstances at the time?

John: Well, a lot would have depended on the amount of time I had left to do anything constructive. I might have worked out that there was enough time to contact my aunt's son by phone, inform him of the situation, and ask him to come and collect her at the airport. Then I might try to contact the airport medical authorities and ask them to look after my aunt until her son arrived to take her home, hoping meanwhile that I might make it to the plane myself on time. Failing that, the only other alternative would be to accept the inevitable and return home, and without liking the loss of my trip, learn to gracefully lump it.

Therapist: Yes, there are other, albeit limited, options you can consider when you are rationally concerned, but no longer panicking about the 'awfulness', of losing your flight. When you are emotionally disturbed about some practical problem – such as coping with the totally unexpected problem of obtaining emergency medication for your aunt, you tend not to see other practicable possibilities there might be of resolving a difficult situation. As a human, you possess a brain capable of both rational and irrational thought. Cultivate your ability to think out rational solutions to everyday problems and hassles, rather than upset yourself over their existence. Many of life's hassles are inevitable, but strongly distressing yourself over them isn't.

John: Yes. I can see that if I want to manage my life's difficulties and stressors without succumbing to distress myself, I'd better work and practise at minimizing my Irrational Beliefs by using the variety of thinking, feeling and behavioural techniques you've taught me. At the same time, I can devise Rational Beliefs and forcefully show myself why they make sense. Then they'll really sink in and become firmly established.

Therapist: I think you're really getting on the right track!

Step 10: Prepare your client to deepen conviction in his or her Rational Beliefs

Your client may now have reached the stage where he has demonstrated a degree of intellectual understanding of his presenting problem. He may also have acknowledged that his weak conviction for Rational Beliefs, while important, doesn't promote change.

Your task now is to help him, during and between therapy sessions, to strengthen his conviction in his Rational Beliefs by disputing his IBs and replacing them with rational alternatives. You can begin by briefly reviewing REBT's three main Insights presented in Chapter 3. You may now reduce your role as an active-directive teacher and encourage your client to work towards becoming his own counsellor.

The more your client practises thinking rationally in relevant life contexts the nearer he will achieve the major philosophic change favoured by REBT. Not all clients will go that far, so don't rigidly — and irrationally! — insist on clients following your own therapeutic goals. When some clients don't work towards achieving a profound philosophic change, you can aim for certain compromises — such as showing them how to change their exaggerated inferences and unwarranted attributions about the behaviour of others. Or, you may help some clients to improve their assertive training or other skills training.[4] Since clients typically subscribe to several Irrational Beliefs, new Adversities and disturbed Consequences will often emerge during the middle phase. These provide an opportunity for clients to try out their newly acquired skills under your watchful guidance and to help them to strengthen their Rational Beliefs. You can encourage your clients to engage in relevant cognitive, emotive and behavioural homework tasks designed to help them to deepen conviction in their Rational Beliefs.

Step 11: Homework assignments

Most REBT counsellors give their clients their first taste of homework assignments by asking them to read specific chapters concerning the application of the ABCs of REBT which they can find in one of the available self-help books such as *A New Guide to Rational Living*, *A Guide to Personal Happiness* and *Think Your Way to Happiness*.[5] You can give clients one of the standard rational emotive behaviour self-help forms which they fill in when they experience some emotional problem in between therapy sessions. They bring this completed form to the next therapy session for review and discussion.

An example of a correctly completed REBT self-help form is shown on pages 65–6.[6] Study it carefully and familiarize yourself with the problems that may arise later with your clients by filling in a few forms yourself. A blank version of the form appears in Appendix 1.

Adequately prepare clients to carry out their homework assignments. Explain that their purpose is to encourage them to practise the new rational ways of thinking and behaving they learn in counselling sessions. Dryden makes these suggestions:[7]

1. Explain why homework is important.
2. Negotiate appropriate assignments that are relevant to your client's problems rather than unilaterally decide them yourself.

3. Ensure that the selected assignments are relevant to your clients achieving their goals.
4. Negotiate assignments which follow from what you have been discussing in the counselling sessions.
5. Agree on *when* clients will carry out assignments and *where* and *how* they will be implemented.
6. Once your clients agree to carry out an assignment, encourage them to rehearse it overtly or in imagery during the session if that is possible. Rehearsals within sessions help to overcome clients' doubts about their ability to carry out their assignments successfully. They help you pinpoint clients' trouble spots (such as anxiety) and may help you deal with Irrational Beliefs that may block the homework.
7. Identify any potential obstacles, such as family involvements, which may interfere with your clients' ability to execute their assignments. Plan how to overcome these obstacles.
8. Be cautious about pushing behaviourally 'flooding' exercises on your client. While these have a certain merit in promoting swift and meaningful modifications to clients' Irrational Belief systems, some clients may balk at carrying out such assignments because they will feel anxious about doing them and will thus avoid doing them. The solution is to agree on an assignment which the client will find challenging, but not overwhelming.[8] This could involve some kind of action the client is not used to and would not feel at ease in executing, but which he would not regard as too difficult or threatening. An example might be assertively requesting a pay rise from an employer, or standing up at a meeting and explaining why he disagrees with the speaker's point of view. We have found it very useful for clients to complete an Assignment Task Sheet (see Appendix 2). This ensures that clients understand the therapeutic reason for the task, and also helps the counsellor to trouble-shoot any obstacles to carrying out the task. You will find an example of a correctly filled out Assignment Task Sheet in Chapter 5, page 74.

Step 12: Check clients' homework assignments

It is important that you check your clients' experiences when they do – or fail to do – their homework. Obtain feedback about what they learned or did not learn from their assignments. You may:

- identify and correct any errors your clients make in carrying out their assignments;
- find out why they avoided doing or failed at their homework. Help them to dispute any Irrational Beliefs which created resistance to their carrying out their assignments;
- if necessary, encourage clients to re-attempt the assignment;
- reinforce your clients' success and urge them to keep making subsequent attempts.

In Appendix 1 of his book *Rational-Emotive Counselling in Action* Dryden identified a number of reasons that clients commonly give for not completing their homework assignments. As he noted, it is better to deal with failures to execute assignments as promptly as feasible.[9]

REBT SELF-HELP FORM

Institute for Rational-Emotive Therapy
45 East 65th Street, New York, NY 10021
(212) 535-0822

(A) ACTIVATING EVENTS, thoughts, or feelings that happened just before I felt emotionally disturbed or acted self-defeatingly: _Make decision about taking a job fairly quickly_

(C) CONSEQUENCE or CONDITION – disturbed feeling or self-defeating behavior – that I produced and would like to change: _Great anxiety_

(B) BELIEFS—Irrational BELIEFS (IBs) leading to my CONSEQUENCE (emotional disturbance or self-defeating behavior). Circle all that apply to these ACTIVATING EVENTS (A).	(D) DISPUTES for each circled IRRATIONAL BELIEF. Examples: "*Why* MUST I do very well? "*Where is it written* that I am a BAD PERSON?" "*Where is the evidence* that I MUST be approved or accepted?"	(E) EFFECTIVE RATIONAL BELIEFS (RBs) to replace my IRRATIONAL BELIEFS (IBs). Examples: "*I'd* PREFER *to do very well but I don't* HAVE TO." "*I am a* PERSON WHO *acted badly, not a BAD PERSON.*" "*There is no evidence that I* HAVE TO *be approved though I would* LIKE *to be.*"
1. I MUST do well or very well! (circled)	_Why MUST I?_	_No reason! – though I'd rather make decisions well._
2. I am a BAD OR WORTHLESS PERSON when I act weakly or stupidly.		
3. I MUST be approved or accepted by people I find important!		
4. I am a BAD, UNLOVABLE PERSON if I get rejected.	_Where is it written that I am a BAD PERSON?_	
5. People must treat me fairly and give me what I NEED!		
6. People who act immorally are undeserving ROTTEN PEOPLE!	_How does an immoral act make you a ROTTEN PERSON?_	
7. People MUST live up to my expectations or it is TERRIBLE!		
8. My life MUST have few major hassles or troubles. (circled)	_Does it really have to have few hassles?_	_No, that would be lovely! But it can easily have all the hassles it really does have!_
9. I CAN'T STAND really bad things or very difficult people!		

10. It's AWFUL or HORRIBLE when major things don't go my way!	How is it horrible?	In no way! It's only a pain in the ass.
11. I CAN'T STAND IT when life is really unfair!		
12. I NEED to be loved by someone who matters to me a lot!		
13. I NEED a good deal of immediate gratification and HAVE TO feel miserable when I don't get it!	Do I need it?	Never. I only strongly want it.
Additional Irrational Beliefs		
14. I should be able to make quick decisions and still always make them well.	Where is this indicated?	Only in my crazy head. I'd better make quick decisions and take the risk of screwing them up.
15.		
16. This job I took must turn out well.	Really? MUST I?	Of course not. If it turns out poorly, too bad! I'll just get another one.

(F) FEELINGS and BEHAVIORS I experienced after arriving at my EFFECTIVE RATIONAL BELIEFS: _Concern but not horror about this quick decision_

I WILL WORK HARD TO REPEAT MY EFFECTIVE RATIONAL BELIEFS FORCE-FULLY TO MYSELF ON MANY OCCASIONS SO THAT I CAN MAKE MYSELF LESS DISTURBED IN THE FUTURE.

Joyce Sichel, PhD and Albert Ellis, PhD
Copyright © 1984 by the Institute for Rational-Emotive Therapy

NOTES

1. Dryden, 1987, 1990a, 1990b, 1995a; Ellis, 1978, 1985a, 1988, 1994a, 1996; Ellis and Becker, 1982; Ellis and Dryden, 1996; Walen, DiGiuseppe and Wessler, 1980; Walen, DiGiuseppe and Dryden, 1992.
2. Dryden, 1995a; see also 1990a, 1990b.
3. Ellis, 1988; Ellis and Becker, 1982; Ellis and Harper, 1975, 1997.
4. Dryden, 1995a.
5. Dryden and Gordon, 1990; Ellis and Becker, 1982; Ellis and Harper, 1975, 1997.
6. Sichel and Ellis, 1984.
7. Dryden, 1990b.
8. Dryden, 1990b, p. 84.
9. Dryden, 1990b.

CHAPTER 5

The Ending Stage of Stress Counselling: Working Towards Termination of Stress Counselling

There is no hard-and-fast dividing line separating the middle stage and the ending stage of counselling. In this final stage, you try to help your client to achieve enduring therapeutic change. When your client shows progress towards this goal and has been responding successfully to your decreased level of directiveness over a period of weeks, you may decide to space out your counselling sessions. Doing so will afford you opportunities to check how well your client is taking the lead in applying the REBT problem-solving method to practise being his own counsellor. During this stage encourage your client to anticipate a variety of future problems and to imagine how he would apply his REBT skills to solving them.

Step 13: Facilitate the working through process

In the working through process, your clients keep forcibly challenging and changing their Irrational Beliefs. As Dryden observes, you enable your client '… to integrate his rational beliefs into his emotional and behavioural repertoire'.[1] This includes cognitive disputing of Irrational Beliefs as well as using emotive and behavioural techniques. This triple-barrelled approach is likely to help clients make a more thorough job of achieving profound philosophic change.

Dealing with relapse

Before ending the counselling relationship with a client, it is advisable to warn him of the possibility of relapse. Explain that relapses are quite normal and that even the brightest of clients will sometimes take two steps forward and one step back. In spite of your client's honest efforts, he may backslide and suffer setbacks. Show him how to avoid denigrating himself when he once again feels and behaves like he is still in the grip of Irrational Beliefs he thought he had left behind ages ago.

Reassure your client that backsliding is par for the course, and that she may be putting herself down for it by telling herself IBs such as 'I *shouldn't* be sliding back like this, especially after all the work I did with my counsellor! I obviously should know better after all my training! What an idiot I am!' If so, she had better get back to basics! – that is, identifying and disputing her Irrational Beliefs and self-downing. Remind her how she once improved. Show her that she can do it again. All she needs is more persistent work and practice to make more enduring progress. Give her a copy to take with her of Albert Ellis's excellent pamphlet *How to Maintain and Enhance Your Rational-Emotive Therapy Gains* which is reproduced in Appendix 4. Your clients will probably find this pamphlet an invaluable aid to maintaining and enhancing their therapeutic gains.

Major counselling techniques in REBT

Many techniques may help clients internalize their newly acquired Rational Beliefs. Be selective in their use and mainly employ those which are likely to help your client to achieve his main therapeutic goals.

As Ellis observes, REBT

> ... looks at the long-range as well as the short-range effects of employing various methods, considers many techniques as more palliative than curative (e.g., cognitive distraction), and tries to emphasize those methods that lead to a profound philosophical and emotional change and that help clients *get* better in addition to *feel* better. It starts most clients off with those REBT methods that usually work best with certain people most of the time; if these fail, it goes on to the use of different methods. It doesn't compulsively choose one or several methods with virtually all clients all of the time, and it fully realizes that some clients, such as those with psychoses or mental retardation, may not be able to use some of the better methods and may have to settle for more palliative techniques.[2]

We note again that because REBT emphasizes the biological as well as the social origins of human disturbance, its practitioners favour the use of medication with certain clients, as well as non-verbal techniques which may include exercise, relaxation and dietary methods.

COGNITIVE TECHNIQUES

1. *Tape-recorded disputing.* Let your client record a disputing sequence on audio-tape. She might, for example, take her IB 'I absolutely *have to* succeed at X or else I'm no good!' and record arguments favouring that Belief. Then she records reasons why her Irrational Belief(s) simply don't make sense and cannot stand up to critical examination. Then she explains why her Rational alternative Belief(s) are more logical, more consistent with reality, and will bring her better results. This technique helps your client convince herself that her Rational Beliefs really do make sense and will help her achieve her goals, whereas her Irrational Beliefs will not. If your client agrees to take this exercise as a homework assignment, check it to see that her rational arguments are powerful enough to overcome her irrational statements.

2. *Rational coping self-statements.* Rational, short coping self-statements can be taped

or written on to 5 inch × 3 inch cards which your client carries around with him and uses to remind himself of rational messages. For example, 'I am not a fool for behaving foolishly, merely a fallible human', 'I never *need* what I *want*', 'Nothing is *awful* in the universe, though many things are inconvenient'. These are best used after your client has learned how to successfully dispute his IBs and has begun to acquire a new effective philosophy at C. Instead of just parroting these statements to himself your client will believe them more strongly if he repeatedly figures out the reasons *why* these statements make sense. Encourage him to come up with other rational self-statements and show you why they make sense and are likely to be more productive.

3. *Referenting.*   Your client makes a list on a card of the *disadvantages* of a dysfunctional behaviour she would like to give up – such as smoking or procrastination. She can also list the *advantages* of giving up her self-defeating behaviour. Reading and thinking about what she has written on her card several times a day helps to sink these rational ideas into her mind and strengthen conviction in her ability to overcome self-defeating habits. As Ellis and Velten note, referenting particularly counters clients' tendencies to dwell only on the immediate 'positive' aspects of their self-defeating behaviour – such as the pleasure they get from puffing a cigarette, or the temporary relief they experience when they procrastinate about carrying out some anxiety-provoking activity.[3] For example, your client can list the following disadvantages associated with smoking: sore throats, increased likelihood of lung cancer, emphysema, high blood pressure, money spent on cigarettes which could be put to better uses, nicotine stains on teeth and fingers, bad breath, offensiveness to other people, and so on. Advantages of stopping smoking can be listed as: better physical and dental health, considerably more money to spend, fresher appearance, less offensive to others. By reviewing (or making references) to these lists daily, clients will often push themselves to give up a bad habit and make themselves more self-disciplined.

4. *Reframing.*   You can help clients to 'reframe', or view differently, some of the 'terrible' things that occur in their lives, and to see that there is often a good side to what they previously viewed as 'awful' or 'horrible'. Thus, they can be shown that being quickly rejected by someone whose acceptance they want can save them much time and energy which they would vainly expend on winning that person's approval.

Again: their being rejected for a job can stimulate them to improve themselves and possibly get an even better job. Clients can also be given the challenge of reframing even very unfortunate Activating Events so as to make themselves feel *only* healthily sorry and disappointed instead of depressed and miserable about them.[4]

5. *Semantic corrections and precision.*   REBT employs some of the principles stated by Alfred Korzybski[5] who originated the philosophy of General Semantics. Korzybski showed that the imprecise use of language often leads to distorted thinking, while at the same time imprecise language often follows from distorted thinking.[6]

REBT shows how the misuse of language helps to sustain and perpetuate Irrational Beliefs through overgeneralizations and invalid identifications. Using REBT, you can show clients how to correct their misleading self-statements – such as 'People *make me* angry when they do stupid things that cause me problems', and to change such statements to 'I *choose* to anger myself over people's mistakes that result in difficulties for me!'[7]

6. *Cognitive homework.* As we stated in Chapter 4, cognitive homework is an important element in the stress counselling process. Clients are given standard self-help forms (available from The Albert Ellis Institute for Rational Emotive Behavior Therapy, New York) to help them write out the ABCs of their disturbances. An example of a correctly filled out self-help form appears on pages 65 and 66 of Chapter 4. Cognitive homework assignments promote efficiency and discourage clients from becoming dependent upon their therapists.[8]

7. *DIBS (Disputing Irrational Beliefs).* DIBS is another example of a structured form of cognitive disputing that is clear, concise and useful.[9] The DIBS form, available from The Albert Ellis Institute for Rational Emotive Behavior Therapy as a pamphlet, consists of six questions which the client asks himself about one of his or her main Irrational Beliefs – such as 'My partner must not treat me unfairly!' The six DIBS questions are:

- What Irrational Belief do I want to dispute and surrender?
- Can I rationally support this Belief?
- What evidence exists of the truth or effectiveness of this Belief?
- What evidence exists of the falseness or ineffectiveness of this Belief?
- What are the worst possible things that could actually happen to me if what I am demanding must not happen actually happens?
- What good things could happen or could I make happen if what I am demanding must not happen actually happens?

Like the REBT self-help forms, DIBS is a useful form to give your clients as part of a negotiated homework assignment. Clients can become enthusiastic about using DIBS when they realize that the 'awful' things they dreamed up amount to nothing more than inconveniences, and that they can constructively deal with these inconveniences. A copy of the DIBS form is shown in Appendix 3. DIBS forms can be obtained from The Albert Ellis Institute for Rational Emotive Behavior Therapy in New York.

8. *Modelling.* You can encourage your client to find models of good behaviour, both in real life and through reading biographies or autobiographies of people who exemplify the principles of rational living. Clients can then follow the rational behaviours of people whom they admire and thereby practise more sensible precepts and actions.

9. *Teaching REBT to others.* As your client progresses in understanding the REBT philosophy, she can often help sink it into her own head and heart by teaching it to friends and relatives. Even if she fails with these others, she may teach it better to herself. However, caution her against over-zealously trying to be an unwanted counsellor to her friends and relations.

10. *Psychoeducational methods.*   It is a fact that people learn by practising what they are taught. Reading the self-help literature and listening to audio and video REBT tapes can appreciably augment your client's in-session learning. The Albert Ellis Institute for Rational Emotive Behavior Therapy in New York produces a regular catalogue listing audio and videotapes as well as many suitable books and pamphlets. Some of the most recommended self-help books are: Ellis, *How to Stubbornly Refuse to Make Yourself Miserable about Anything – Yes, Anything!*; Ellis and Harper, *A New Guide to Rational Living*; Ellis and Becker, *A Guide to Personal Happiness*; Ellis and Knaus, *Overcoming Procrastination*; Hauck, *Overcoming the Rating Game*.[10] Books published in the UK by Sheldon Press, London, include: Dryden, *Overcoming Guilt*; Dryden, *Overcoming Anger*; Dryden and Gordon, *Think Your Way to Happiness*; Dryden and Gordon, *Beating the Comfort Trap*.[11] These can be obtained from the Centre for REBT, London.

11. *Cognitive distractions.*   Sometimes, clients may be too disturbed to be able to undertake effective disputing of their Irrational Beliefs. In such cases, cognitive distraction techniques may be used to help allay their disturbed feelings and help them later come round to carrying out effective Disputing. Distraction methods include biofeedback, progressive relaxation, Yoga and meditation, and other methods described in Chapter 6.

EMOTIVE TECHNIQUES

REBT holds that people's dysfunctional thoughts, feelings and behaviours are often deep-rooted and held on to firmly and strongly. Therefore, to reduce them, clients had better work hard at changing their irrational thinking, but also use a number of REBT's vigorous evocative-emotive and behavioural techniques. You can use the following evocative-emotive techniques not just for your clients' immediate benefit but also to help them make and maintain a profound and lasting philosophic change:

1. *Shame attacking.*   When clients do something they consider wrong, stupid, incompetent or immoral, they very often make themselves feel thoroughly ashamed, or guilty, depressed or worthless. Shame-attacking exercises are designed to help them to minimize their self-downing feelings of humiliation. You show your clients how they create self-depreciation by insisting that, first, they *absolutely must* do well, especially in public. Second, if they act stupidly or ineptly in front of others (as they believe they *must not*) they define themselves as worthless individuals.

To do shame-attacking exercises you help clients to think of some act or behaviour that they consider shameful, ridiculous, stupid, embarrassing or humiliating, but which would be unlikely to land them in serious trouble if they actually did it. Having picked one such act, clients actually do it at least once but preferably several times in full view of friends, relatives or members of the public.

Typical exercises carried out by clients include: (a) refusing to tip a waiter or cab driver who has given you poor service; (b) expressing dislike for the behaviour of someone you know when you are afraid to speak up; (c) expressing a tender or loving compliment to someone you know, for fear that you will act awkwardly. Your clients can also deliberately carry out acts that others will consider silly or crazy, such as getting on a subway train or a bus during a busy period and shouting out the stops at the top of their voice – and staying on the train, or bus!

Shame-attacking exercises help clients convince themselves that *nothing* is really shameful, embarrassing or humiliating, unless they *think* it is. Instead of putting themselves down as they perform their exercises, clients can tell themselves 'I'm obviously acting stupidly in public, but that doesn't make me a stupid or worthless person!'

If you have not already done so, it is a useful and educative experience to carry out some shame-attacking exercises yourself before giving them to your clients to do. As you carry out these exercises you may first experience intense feelings of shame and embarrassment. Don't run away from these feelings. Stay in the situation and really feel them. See what you are telling yourself to create these feelings. Then you dispute and change your self-downing Irrational Beliefs that create your 'shameful' feelings and overcome them. Shame-attacking exercises are an excellent form of *in vivo* desensitization. For you and your clients it can become one of the best ways of revealing and overcoming self-depreciating Beliefs.

2. *Risk-taking exercises.* In risk-taking exercises, you encourage clients to push themselves to undertake some activity they would like to engage in (such as taking the initiative to speak to an attractive member of the opposite sex) but which they are currently refraining from doing because they consider it 'too risky'. They thus learn that the outcome they feared is not at all 'awful' or 'terrible' and that they can easily handle it. Repeated engaging in some feared activity, such as public speaking, may not only help a client to overcome his awfulizing about the possibility of doing it badly. It may also tend to make him a better public speaker simply through practice.[12]

An illustrative example of risk-taking and shame-attacking. Tim was fond of modern dancing and he had been attending dancing classes for some considerable time. In class Tim happily danced with any of the women at his own level, but when he went to public dances he avoided asking any woman to dance whom he considered better than himself.

At the same time, Tim felt frustrated; he wanted to improve his own dancing by dancing with better partners but was ashamed to ask. He felt he would be 'imposing' on them and that they would look down on him if he danced poorly.

Even when a woman approached him and asked him to dance, Tim would make up some excuse and refuse the invitation. His frustration, of course, increased. Tim mentioned his problem to an REBT counsellor and their dialogue went as follows:

> *Counsellor:* Let's suppose that you did approach one of these better dancers and asked her to dance with you. What do you imagine would happen?
>
> *Tim:* Well, when she found out that I wasn't very good she'd feel she had wasted her time dancing with me. She would think that I had some nerve asking someone at her level to dance with someone like me who is practically a beginner. Or, she might even refuse me outright.
>
> *Counsellor:* Yes, some women might respond in either of these ways, others might not. But suppose they all responded negatively to you when you ask them to dance with you. How would you feel?

Tim: Pretty embarrassed and ashamed, I should say. Wouldn't everybody feel the same in that situation?

Counsellor: Not necessarily. If somebody doesn't like the way you dance, or just doesn't fancy dancing with you, that is their view, their taste. They are entitled to their likes and dislikes. But why put yourself down – which is what you do when you feel ashamed or embarrassed?

Tim: So, I suppose I'm really agreeing with their negative evaluation. Is that it?

Counsellor: Well, they may be evaluating you negatively, but the chances are that they are only putting down your *dancing ability*. It is *you* who are rating *you* negatively. You are saying to yourself 'These women think my dancing is no good, therefore *I* am no good'. Isn't that what you are telling yourself?

Tim: Yeah, I suppose so. And then I avoid asking them to dance with me in order not to embarrass them.

Counsellor: No, you avoid dancing with them in order not to embarrass *you*. They're not embarrassed, *you* are!

Tim: OK, how do I act in future so as not to feel embarrassed and ashamed when I dance with one of these better dancers, or when I get turned down?

Counsellor: First, by convincing yourself 'I strongly *prefer* to dance well with any prospective partner I am likely to meet, but *I don't have to*'. Second, forcing yourself to ask better dancers to dance with you will provide you with the opportunity to identify and dispute the nonsense you are telling yourself when you feel embarrassed. Such as: 'They *mustn't* reject me or criticize the way I dance because that would mean I'm no good!'

You can even learn to welcome constructive criticism if you get it because that's how you can improve and raise your own level of dancing ability. So, the next time you attend one of those public dances, go right up and ask at least six of the good dancers to dance with you. And as you do so, remind yourself of your Rational Belief: 'I would very much *like* to dance well with this person but I don't *have to*. If I fail and disappoint her, and perhaps get criticized, it isn't the end of the world. It's merely unfortunate, and I can accept myself with my lack of experience. Every time I dance is a potential learning experience. The more I keep trying, the more I can learn, and the sooner I can reach the standard I'm aiming for.' Wouldn't it be good for you to try that kind of risk-taking exercise?

Tim agreed that it would help, and he filled in an Assignment Task Sheet (see page 74).

On his next counselling session, Tim could hardly wait to tell his counsellor what had happened.

Counsellor: Well, Tim, how did your shame-attacking and risk-taking exercise work out?

Tim: Well, I did just what you said. One woman refused me pointblank when I asked her to dance. Another woman walked off the floor in the middle of a dance and left me standing there.

Counsellor: How did you feel about being refused?

Tim: Well, I took the rejection in my stride. I was half expecting it, anyway. One just said 'No thank you'. I didn't feel put down, I just said 'OK, maybe another time', and then I asked this other woman to dance.

ASSIGNMENT TASK SHEET

Name: _Tim_   **Date:** _19/10/95_   **Negotiated with:** _Helen_

Agreed task: _Go to the next public dance run by my dance club and ask 6 partners whom I rate as superior to myself in dancing expertise to dance with me at least once. If I feel embarrassed about asking these good dancers to dance with me in case they refuse or criticize my dancing, I will challenge my negative thoughts and Irrational Beliefs about myself and replace them with the Rational Beliefs and coping statements I learned during my counselling sessions. Then I will force myself to approach the 6 good dancers I have picked out and dance with each one!_

The therapeutic purpose(s) of the task: _To enable me the next time I'm in a similar situation, to ask anyone I want to dance with me regardless of how good they are, because I can convince myself that being rejected or criticized can never be 'awful' or 'embarrassing', but only frustrating and disappointing. Moreover, by risking negative reactions from partners with superior dance skills. I can learn not only to refuse to put myself down, or to feel embarrassed, but I can improve my own dancing through accepting criticism of my technique without taking the criticism personally._

Obstacles to carrying out the task – what obstacles, if any, stand in your way of completing this task and how you can overcome them:

1 _I might still cop out of doing my assignment, especially if all the dancers present look pretty good. But I can overcome my irrational fears by forcing myself to act against them while reminding myself_
2 _as I do so of my coping statements as well as the penalty I will incur if I fail to do the assignment. I can also remind myself that the sooner I face my fears and do the assignment in full, the_
3 _sooner I will feel better and begin to get better. The longer I put off <u>risking</u> the longer I'll go on <u>suffering</u>!_

Penalty: _If I fail to carry out my assignment as agreed I will donate £10 to each of the three main political parties in this country._

Reward: _If I carry out my assignment correctly I will reward myself by listening for one hour to my favourite jazz CD or jazz dance video._

                                        Signed: _Tim_

Counsellor: And how did you feel when this other person you asked to dance just walked off and left you standing in the middle of the floor?

Tim: All right, actually. I was more surprised than sorry. She just suddenly excused herself and walked off. I thought it was poor etiquette because you're not supposed to do that except for some really serious reason, like suddenly feeling ill, or something like that. So I said 'Are you feeling all right?' and she just said 'Yes, I'm OK' and walked off the floor. I felt disappointed because I was beginning to enjoy myself.

Counsellor: So far so good. You seem to have coped quite well. One rejection and one walkout and you were still refusing to put yourself down.

Tim: No, and listen to this. Like you suggested, I danced with four other good dancers after that episode, and I even enjoyed it. And guess what? The last one of the four I danced with made it seem so easy for me that I looked like a far better dancer than I actually am. She guided me through interesting steps I hadn't done before; she was really good, this woman, real topnotch. I had seen her dancing before in competitions and she had a regular partner and they won prizes. That was the level she was at. So I said to her as the music stopped 'You know, it makes such a difference to me having a really good partner to dance with!' Well do you know what she did? Turning towards me as I said that, she gave my hand a firm squeeze, and with a beautiful smile on her face, said 'We must dance together again some other time!'

Counsellor: So you felt good about it!

Tim: Felt good! I felt over the moon!

Counsellor: Ah! But suppose every single one of these good dancers had rejected you. How would you have felt then? You find that not a single one of them will dance with you. How would you have felt about that?

Tim: Well, I would have been very disappointed.

Counsellor: Only disappointed?

Tim: Yes. Before, I took it too seriously. I took refusal as a kind of personal putdown. And I thought those good dancers whom I admired and really wanted to dance with would consider I had a bit of a cheek to even ask them to dance with the likes of me. I mean, I'm nowhere near their level of expertise, so I thought they would think 'How boring!' once they started to dance with me and discovered I wasn't up to their standard. Not that they ever came right out and said so, but I thought they must be thinking it!

Counsellor: So, you inferred that certain partners took a poor view of your dancing ability. Then you took their presumed low opinion of your dancing prowess and jumped from 'They don't think much of my dancing' to 'So they don't think much of me!' Then because you agreed with their presumed low evaluation, you felt ashamed and consequently avoided approaching those women whom you rated superior dancers in case they rejected you and thereby confirmed your low opinion of yourself.

Tim: Yes, I see now how self-defeating that was. I was rating *me*, my totality, on the basis of one particular aspect of me, namely my ability on the dance floor. Even if my dancing ability is deficient, that doesn't amount to, or equal, my entire personhood. I see now that even if I got rejected every time by good dancers, that doesn't say anything about me as a person. It might mean that certain people prefer to dance only with partners who have reached a certain level of proficiency. That is their right. They don't have to dance with anybody who comes along and asks them. They can choose whom they wish to dance with. Or they might have preferences for certain partners, people they know well, for example. There could be all sorts of reasons for people's preferences when it comes to finding partners for dancing, or for anything else for that matter. People are entitled to their preferences, their prejudices, and their likes and dislikes.

Counsellor: Right. Acting against your fears is important. Going out and doing what you were irrationally afraid to do is one of the best ways of confronting your embarrassment and of revealing the shame-creating Irrational Beliefs that underlie it. By vigorously disputing your Irrational Beliefs *at the same time* as you force yourself to act against them, you can overcome them and give up your feelings of shame and embarrassment. If you practise thinking and acting against your self-defeating feelings, regardless of what form they take, they will eventually lose their ability to hold you back from doing what you want to do, and no longer be a problem to you.

As the above dialogue demonstrates, whatever form of recreation you enjoy, you can easily cancel out its potential benefits if you make yourself stressed by the irrational demands you make upon yourself and other people. For example, we have met people devoted to the game of bridge who can become extremely angry and upset at what they consider to be their partner's poor tactics or bad play. Some people become so emotionally distressed that they refuse to speak to their partners or to the other players. We know of a long-standing friendship that was broken because of a dispute over who was to blame for a particular game being lost.

Enjoyment of some sport or recreational activity is fine. It is one way of reducing stress. Ironically, activities which people choose to help them relax often end up as 'stressors'. You can help your clients avoid this if they practise monitoring their thoughts and feelings, especially in competitive activities, and learn to identify and challenge the absolutistic musts, shoulds and oughts that often sabotage their 'enjoyments'.

3. *Self-disclosure exercises.* You can ask clients, especially in therapy groups and workshops, to reveal some secret they would least like someone else to know about. Or, ask them to express themselves in a way they would consider risky. Ensure confidentiality, however, so that group members won't reveal secrets, or a risky or 'shameful' piece of information to others outside the group. You don't want to see clients being fired from their jobs or expelled from a school or club!

Self-disclosure can often encourage others to disclose their own secrets and evasions and thereby help to improve interpersonal relations. Combine self-revealing exercises with REBT's cognitive disputing and anti-awfulizing techniques to help clients cope with others' possible negative reactions. Show them that they never have to put themselves down because of criticism.

4. *Role-playing.* This can teach your clients how to go about carrying out some action which they are afraid to perform. One example is where the client is about to

go for a job interview. Another is where the client wishes to learn how to approach members of the same or opposite sex.

In performing a role-playing exercise, you – or possibly a group member, if appropriate – play the part of the job interviewer, for example, or the person the client wishes to encounter. The client plays himself and speaks as he imagines he should speak in order to impress the other person were they in a real life situation. From the feedback he gets from the therapist or group on how he came across in the interaction, the client learns how he could improve his manner, style of speaking and so on, and thus improve his chances of doing better the next time a similar kind of encounter occurs.

In doing role-playing your clients may realize that the event they are rehearsing is not really as formidable or risky as they think it is, and that even if they do badly or fail to get the result they want, it isn't the end of the world, nor is it the last chance they will ever have. In the cognitive disputing that accompanies the execution of these exercises, clients can focus on the *self-rating* and *always and never* aspects of their Irrational Beliefs and convince themselves that even when they perform poorly they don't have to rate themselves at all, but only their performances. They can convince themselves that this is unlikely to be the last chance they will ever have of trying for what they want, and that by working persistently to improve their interpersonal skills, they will have a better chance of correcting their faults and of succeeding in future. While doing uncomfortable role-plays clients get an opportunity to dispute discomfort-related beliefs, such as 'I *must* feel comfortable about doing this exercise' or 'I *can't stand* the uncertainty of not knowing what will happen'.[13]

5. *Rational-emotive imagery (REI)*.   Pioneered by Maultsby and modified by Ellis for use in REBT, REI is a technique designed to promote emotive insight while vividly imagining some disturbance-provoking situation at A.[14] In Chapter 4 we gave you one example of the Ellis version of the use of REI.

In the Maultsby version of REI, the client first imagines something unpleasant or disadvantageous has happened, or is likely to happen to him. He then makes himself feel anxious, hostile or disturbed about his image. Then he looks for the Irrational Beliefs he is holding that create his disturbed feelings and he works hard on changing these Beliefs by vigorously disputing them and replacing them with Rational Beliefs.

Next, the client strongly pictures himself disbelieving these Irrational Beliefs and instead pictures himself feeling and acting in accordance with his new Rational Beliefs. Instead of feeling anxious or hostile, he pictures himself replacing these unhealthy negative feelings with healthier feelings of concern or displeasure.

Behaviourally, the client can imagine himself looking for better solutions to his unpleasant Activating experience at A, and fully accepting himself no matter how poorly he may have behaved in his imagination.

6. *Reverse role-playing*.   Here you adopt the role of devil's advocate and rigidly hold one of the client's Irrational Beliefs, while she tries to talk you out of this IB. In presenting irrational arguments to your client, you are inviting her to refute your arguments – and at the same time defend her rational arguments which are really her own. By this means you can identify and help correct weak points in your client's

thinking. You can also let your client present a Rational Belief, try to talk her forcefully out of it, and give her practice in effectively defending it.

7. *Forceful self-dialogues.* This is essentially a dialogue your client has with himself. Your client makes an audiotape describing and attempting to justify his Irrational Beliefs. This is his *irrational voice.* He then vigorously Disputes his IBs and you (and others) listen to see how forceful his Disputing is and if he really has given up his IBs.[15] Examples of forceful dialogues can be studied in *Rational-Emotive Therapy with Alcoholics and Substance Abusers* by Ellis, McInerney, DiGiuseppe and Yeager, and in *Beating the Comfort Trap* by Dryden and Gordon.[16] Listen carefully to your client's tape to make sure his Disputing is sufficiently powerful to convince him that his IBs are untenable.

8. *Use of humour and paradoxical intention.* In REBT, humour is used to encourage your clients to see the absurd or amusing aspects of their Irrational Beliefs. As Ellis has observed, disturbed people tend to take life too seriously and frequently lose their sense of humour. By helping clients to laugh at some of their irrational ideas and behaviours, you can interrupt their over-serious way of viewing themselves and the world and help them to surrender some of their Irrational Beliefs and self-defeating behaviours.[17] When using humour, direct it at your client's ideas rather than at the client himself. Ellis and Abrahms show how the case we discussed above in which Tim feared rejection by superior dancers could have been humorously Disputed as follows:

> And of course, if you dance poorly, everyone on the dance floor will stop and guffaw, do nothing else but think about you all night, and keep remembering your crummy dancing for the next forty years. Right?[18]

Use humorous interventions sparingly and only when you have achieved a good working therapeutic alliance, and you feel confident that there is little danger that she will take it amiss if you good-humouredly poke fun at some of her irrational ideas.

Ellis has written a number of rational humorous songs which clients are encouraged to sing at times when they make themselves unduly disturbed. Rational humorous songs are also a regular feature in REBT workshops and presentations and are a good way of getting participants to 'lighten up' and take an active part in the proceedings.[19]

9. *Time projection.* You can use this technique with clients who keep dreaming up doom and gloom. For example, your client may view it as 'terrible' if he possibly loses the one surviving member of his family, his only sister, who is ill with cancer. You can challenge your client's awfulizing by temporarily going along with it while asking him to imagine what his life would be like at increasing intervals in the future after the dreaded event has occurred. By asking him to visualize a time in the future – say, in a year from now – and by including positive suggestions and images of his then doing things that he has enjoyed in the past, you may help him see that the feared happening need not be as 'terrible' as he makes out, and that he can still lead a happy life. You may use time projection in cases where a client's anxiety or depression is triggered by some important life event, such as job loss or divorce.[20]

10. *Unconditional self-acceptance.*   When you give your clients unconditional self-acceptance (USA) you fully accept *all* of them as very fallible humans. You don't necessarily love or like them or their *behaviours* but you forgive *them* with their 'sins'. By considering *them* worthy of help and enjoyment, no matter what they *do*, you serve as a good model for their thoroughly accepting themselves.

Watch it, however! Your clients may accept themselves mainly because *you* – and not really *they* – do. But this is *conditional* self-acceptance. To bring these clients round to *un*conditionally and fully accepting themselves as 'deserving' to stay alive and be happy, you usually have to *teach* them to choose unconditional self-acceptance. This means showing them why it is inefficient to rate themselves in any way, although they may usefully rate their deeds and traits in terms of their goals.[21]

11. *Other emotive techniques.*   In your REBT counselling you can use a number of emotive-evocative techniques including self-disclosure, stories, aphorisms, mottoes, analogies and metaphors. REBT therapists find it useful to build up a fund of such stories, for use on appropriate occasions. You thereby convey rational messages and enhance your client's Disputing.[22]

BEHAVIOURAL TECHNIQUES

Sadly enough, once people keep victimizing themselves with irrational thoughts and self-defeating feelings, they tend to continue their neurotic behaviour even when they realize how foolish it is. We are habit-forming creatures, who can learn and practise good, healthy life-enhancing habits, as well as over-eating, compulsive drinking, procrastinating and other destructive addictions. While some unhealthy habits are socially learned, others probably stem from our biological tendencies for self-abuse.[23]

REBT therefore includes a number of active behavioural methods of facilitating cognitive and emotional change. Being constructivist, it uses the interactive nature of thoughts, feelings and actions.[24] Some of the most common REBT behavioural techniques you can use to promote client change are the following:

1. In vivo *desensitization.*   Because, as John Dewey said, we learn by doing, REBT favours *in vivo* over imaginal desensitization to help clients overcome their long-standing anxieties and phobias.[25] Thus, you can often work out with clients assignments to do what they are most afraid to do and to do it many times, implosively. Typical assignments might include speaking in public, upholding an unpopular view amongst friends or colleagues, encountering potential sex-love partners, and undertaking important job interviews. You can often use flooding over more gradual methods to help some of your clients desensitize themselves faster and more thoroughly to the 'horrors' they imagine they will face. Implosive methods also may encourage clients to overcome their LFT more quickly than more gradual desensitization. In a paper on popular behaviour therapy techniques Ellis proposes that gradual exposure methods may inadvertently reinforce the client's LFT by encouraging him to believe 'I must avoid making myself uncomfortable at all costs'.[26] Sometimes, however, you may persuade clients who find implosive desensitization too 'overwhelming' to carry out an assignment that is challenging and uncomfortable, but not overwhelmingly so.[27]

2. *Anti-procrastination exercises.* Procrastination often stems from discomfort disturbance. Clients easily convince themselves that certain tasks are 'too difficult' or 'too uncomfortable' for them to tolerate, and that they *shouldn't* have to put up with such discomfort. They then avoid doing those uncomfortable tasks, or put them off for as long as they can. You can use anti-procrastination exercises to show your clients that when they expose themselves to an 'unbearable' task they can prove to themselves that they can indeed deal with discomfort and accomplish what they are avoiding. Pushing your clients to overcome their procrastination helps attack their discomfort anxiety and increase their frustration tolerance.[28]

3. *Remaining in 'awful' situations.* REBT practitioners often encourage clients to remain temporarily in uncomfortable situations, stop viewing them as 'awful', and then decide whether it is worth staying. Suppose, for example, you have a client who has been suddenly pushed into undertaking new responsibility and is and feels very stressed because he now fears he will handle his colleagues poorly. He feels anxious about messing up his job and he often flies into a rage over his colleagues' constant criticism and their attempts to usurp activities that he believes are now his own responsibility. He sleeps badly and he suspects he is developing a stomach ulcer.

You would first try to help this client overcome his distress by finding and reducing his IBs. Then, as he gets himself into a healthier frame of mind, you would encourage him to take some practical steps to solve his work problem – such as asking the management to set out clear written guidelines delineating his responsibilities. If you do not help him first resolve his overly stressed feelings he is liable to take his anxiety to any future job problems he encounters.[29]

4. *Relaxation methods.* Various relaxation techniques are used in REBT, mainly in an ancillary or palliative role, to help clients relax as they are directly attacking the core ideas underlying their feelings of stress. Some of the more popular of these techniques will be described in Chapter 6.

5. *Reinforcement and penalization.* When clients experience difficulty in undertaking challenging homework assignments, you can collaborate with them on a system of rewards and penalties designed to encourage their implementing their homework. Rewards and penalties are individually tailored to clients who are asked what they really enjoy doing. The performance of this pleasurable activity is then made contingent upon their doing and completing their agreed upon homework assignment.

When clients fail to carry out their assignments, they can apply a penalty to themselves. You agree with them beforehand on penalties such as cleaning the kitchen or bathroom, or getting up in the morning an hour earlier than usual. If that isn't severe enough a more obnoxious penalty may be employed, such as their burning a £50 note, or contributing a sum of money to some political or religious cause they detest. Sometimes a combination of rewards and penalties works best with some clients. As Ellis and Becker note, 'The use of immediate rewards or reinforcements for doing difficult homework assignments and the employment of strict, quickly enforced penalties for not doing them works very well with REBT clients'.[30]

6. *Response prevention.*   This is a technique which may be used with clients suffering from obsessions and compulsions. They cut them down behaviourally while also Disputing the Irrational Beliefs underlying them.[31] See also Chapter 8 for a more detailed discussion of treating obsessive-compulsive behaviours.

7. *Medication.*   Clients severely afflicted with emotional-behavioural problems may often benefit from medication, including antidepressants, lithium and other drugs targeted at specific disorders. As Ellis notes, you can encourage these treatments while also helping your clients work first on their LFT so as to increase the likelihood that they will actually follow the medication procedures prescribed for them.[32]

8. *Stimulus control.*   While REBT practitioners almost always try to help clients to change their self-disturbing cognitions and evaluations about their unfortunate Activating Experiences, your clients sometimes can control stimuli that tend to trigger self-defeating behaviour. You can, for example, show clients with overeating problems how to remove tempting foods from their habitats. At the same time, you can help them learn about health, nutrition and to Dispute their Irrational Beliefs, such as 'I *must* have immediate gratification when I crave something to eat and I *can't bear* the frustration when I am deprived of it'.[33] Chapter 8 will be found helpful for those who require information on the treatment of more serious disorders such as bulimia and anorexia.

DEALING WITH OBSTACLES TO CHANGE

As you and your client work towards termination, look for evidence that he has made significant progress in overcoming the problems for which he originally sought therapy, and also is generalizing his REBT knowledge to dealing with other kinds of self-depreciation, rage and low frustration tolerance. Hopefully he now takes the lead in exploring new problems, and anticipates dealing with future difficulties.

However, as you work towards helping your client to become her own counsellor unexpected obstacles may arise. Resistance to change can emerge, often in subtle ways. The phenomenon of resistance justifies a book in itself, and indeed Ellis authored a book on the subject, *Overcoming Resistance: Rational-Emotive Therapy with Difficult Clients*, which we recommend.[34] You will also find a helpful discussion of common aspects of resistance in Chapter 8 of this book. Some frequently encountered reasons for resistance to change include these:

1. *Low frustration tolerance (LFT).*   You can often attribute resistance to clients' low tolerance of frustration. They fail to follow through on their earlier successes because they believe the effort required of them is too onerous. Typical IBs you will encounter here are 'Change *must not* be difficult' or 'I *should not* have to work so hard in counselling'.[35] Check out such possible LFT philosophies and help resistors to challenge and change them.

2. *Intellectual insight alone is enough.*   Some clients will acknowledge that REBT makes a lot of sense but become more adept at explaining than applying it in action.

Some clients believe that if they read enough books and listen to enough REBT audiotapes, somehow rational philosophies will automatically sink in and all will be well. Point out to such clients that REBT doesn't *itself* work. They have to *make* it work by actively Disputing their Irrational Beliefs *and* by *acting* against them.

Remind resistant clients of Insight no. 3: They'd better make building and maintaining a high level of emotional health a top priority for the rest of their life. There are no quick fixes!

3. *Combat Irrational Beliefs vigorously.* Remember that the 'softly, softly' approach often doesn't work here. Ellis, and Yankura and Dryden, have argued that since clients often adhere to their Irrational Beliefs with considerable tenacity, even after they realize that these beliefs lie at the root of their emotional and behavioural problems, you'd better teach them how to attack their Irrational Beliefs with force and energy.[36]

4. *Attack Irrational Beliefs frequently.* Newcomers to REBT tend to Dispute IBs in parrot fashion. They see that their IBs don't make sense, but they 'see' it only lightly. The more *frequently* your clients attack their IBs, the sooner they will acquire deep conviction that they are unrealistic, illogical and thereby weaken obstacles to change.

5. *Add persistence to disputing.* Assaults on Irrational Beliefs require *persistence*. Most clients' IBs have a long history, and their tenaciously held beliefs will not be dismantled in a week or two. By adding persistence to the vigour and frequency of their disputing tehniques, your clients are more likely to make real and enduring gains.

6. *Cognitive-emotive dissonance.* 'The neurotic fear of being a phoney' can obstruct change. As clients work towards change and begin to make real progress, they sometimes feel 'unnatural'. Believing they must feel 'natural' at all times, they tend to think 'This isn't me, I'm not really me!' They fear they are losing their identity.

You can say to them 'Let's assume that you have been out of condition for some time. When you begin an exercise programme, you may feel strange at first. "This isn't me!" But as you persist and gradually improve your physique, you will begin to feel quite at home with your new exercise regime.' Suggest to your clients that they print on a 5 inch × 3 inch card the words '*Persistence is the key*' and that they carry the card around with them and read it several times daily to remind themselves of the value of sticking to their programme for change and becoming 'a new person'.

NOTES

1. Dryden, 1990b, p. 65.
2. Ellis, 1990a, pp. 85–6.
3. Ellis and Velten, 1992.
4. Ellis, 1988, 1996.
5. Korzybski, 1933.

6. Ellis and Becker, 1982.
7. Ellis and Harper, 1975, 1997.
8. Yankura and Dryden, 1990.
9. Ellis, 1974a; Ellis and Harper, 1975.
10. Ellis, 1988; Ellis and Becker, 1982; Ellis and Harper, 1975, 1997; Ellis and Knaus, 1977; Hauck, 1991.
11. Dryden, 1994b, 1996; Dryden and Gordon, 1990a, 1993b.
12. Ellis and Dryden, 1990; Palmer and Dryden, 1995; Yankura and Dryden, 1990, 1994.
13. Dryden, 1987, p. 133.
14. Ellis, 1993a; Maultsby and Ellis, 1974.
15. Ellis, 1993b.
16. Dryden and Gordon, 1993; Ellis, McInerney, DiGiuseppe and Yeager, 1988.
17. Ellis, 1977a, 1977b.
18. Ellis and Abrahms, 1978.
19. Ellis, 1977a, 1977b, 1987a.
20. Palmer and Dryden, 1995.
21. Ellis, 1994a, 1996; Ellis, McInerney, DiGiuseppe and Yeager, 1988.
22. Ellis, 1994a, 1996; Ellis and Dryden, 1987, 1991; Ellis and Yeager, 1989.
23. Ellis, 1976, 1994a, 1996.
24. Ellis, 1962, 1990a, 1991a, 1994a.
25. Ellis, 1983b; Ellis and Abrahms, 1978.
26. Ellis, 1983.
27. Dryden, 1990b, p. 84.
28. Ellis and Knaus, 1977.
29. Ellis, 1985a, 1988; Ellis and Abrahms, 1978.
30. Ellis and Becker, 1982, p. 58.
31. Ellis, 1985a; Ellis and Velten, 1992.
32. Ellis, 1985a; Ellis and Abrahms, 1978.
33. Ellis and Abrahms, 1978, pp. 115, 117.
34. Ellis, 1985a.
35. Dryden, 1990b.
36. Ellis, 1979b, 1985, 1991a, 1994a, 1996; Yankura and Dryden, 1990.

CHAPTER 6

Additional Techniques for Stress Counselling with REBT

Theoretically, any of the methods of psychotherapy can be used by rational emotive behaviour therapists as long as they do not promote irrational thinking or are self-defeating. REBT practitioners would also be reluctant to use methods which help people *only* to feel better, and not to get better. But there are no rigid or absolute rules in this matter.[1] From time to time you will see individual clients that you are fairly sure will be capable of making only very limited gains from REBT – such as those with psychosis and severe personality disorders. You may then mainly use palliative methods, including support and reassurance, changing the person's environment, or directly instructing them on how to run their lives. With the majority of clients, however, you can quite often use some of the more important aspects of REBT, such as cognitive disputing, REI and *in vivo* homework assignments.

As Ellis notes, '... almost all of the psychotherapies (as well as, even, the drug therapies) are informative, instructive, persuasive, and suggestive, and most of them include large elements of focusing, imagining, interpretation, and covert or overt philosophizing, all of which are highly cognitive processes'.[2] So whatever treatments you employ, unless your clients are exceptionally deficient, they will *think* about the treatments they are undergoing. If you bear in mind the enormous part that cognition plays in human affairs, you can use scores of cognitive methods to alleviate stress disorders. Let us now add some of those we have discussed previously.

Cognitive distractions

You can use various kinds of distractions to help clients to temporarily deal with distress.

Progressive relaxation was first introduced by Edmund Jacobson and subsequently refined and used by Joseph Wolpe and Arnold Lazarus as a reciprocal inhibition method.[3] The entire procedure takes approximately 20 minutes and is useful for tense clients who are suffering from generalized and specific anxiety and a number of physical ailments, including hypertension.

To illustrate how this technique is used, the following quote from Palmer and Dryden describes part of the relaxation of the arms:

> Settle back as comfortably as you can. Let yourself relax to the best of your ability
> .... Now, as you relax like that, clench your right fist, just clench your fist tighter
> and tighter, and study the tension as you do so. Keep it clenched and feel the
> tension in your right fist, hand, forearm ... and now relax. Let the fingers of your
> right hand become loose, and observe the contrast in your feelings.... Now, let
> yourself go and try to become more relaxed all over.... Once more, clench your
> right fist tight ... hold it, and notice the tension again.... Now let go, relax; your
> fingers straighten out, and you notice the difference once more ... [and so on].

However, as Palmer and Dryden have shown, care needs to be taken with clients with hypertension and high blood pressure to ensure that the muscle-tensing parts of the relaxation procedures do not dangerously raise their blood pressure.[4]

Multimodal relaxation is a method devised by Stephen Palmer and is indicated for all individuals wishing to learn a relatively safe relaxation technique. Palmer gives details on this method that provides several relaxation techniques for participants in stress management, anxiety management and group relaxation courses.[5]

The complete multimodal relaxation script is reprinted below from *Multimodal Techniques: Relaxation and Hypnosis*, pp. 17–23, by kind permission of the author.

The MRM script

If you could make yourself as comfortable as possible on your chair

PAUSE
and if you would just like to close your eyes

PAUSE
As you do this exercise, if you feel any odd feelings such as tingling sensations, light headedness, or whatever, then this is quite normal. If you open your eyes then these feelings will go away. If you carry on with the relaxation exercise usually the feelings will disappear anyway

PAUSE
If you would like to listen to the noises outside the room first of all

LONG PAUSE
And now listen to the noises inside the room

PAUSE
You may be aware of yourself breathing

PAUSE
These noises will come and go probably throughout this session and you can choose to let them just drift over your mind and choose to ignore them if you so wish

PAUSE
Now keeping your eyelids closed and without moving your head, I would like you to look upwards, your eyes closed, just look upwards

PAUSE (NB: If participants wear contact lenses then they can remove them before the exercise or not look upwards)
Notice the feeling of tiredness

PAUSE
And relaxation

PAUSE
In your eye muscles

PAUSE
Now let your eyes drop back down

PAUSE
Notice the tiredness and the relaxation in those muscles of your eyes

PAUSE
Let the feeling now travel down your face to your jaw, just relax your jaw

LONG PAUSE
Now relax your tongue

PAUSE
Let the feeling of relaxation slowly travel up over your face to the top of your head

PAUSE
To the back of your head

LONG PAUSE
Then slowly down through the neck muscles

PAUSE
And down to your shoulders

LONG PAUSE
Now concentrate on relaxing your shoulders, just let them drop down

PAUSE
Now let that feeling of relaxation in your shoulders slowly travel down your right arm, down through the muscles, down through your elbow, down through your wrist, to your hand, right down to your finger tips

LONG PAUSE
Let the feeling of relaxation now in your shoulders slowly travel down your left arm, down through your muscles, down through your elbow, down through your wrist, to your hand, right down to your finger tips

LONG PAUSE
And let that feeling of relaxation now in your shoulders slowly travel down your chest, right down to your stomach

PAUSE
Just concentrate now on your breathing

PAUSE
Notice that every time as you breathe out you feel more

PAUSE
And more relaxed

LONG PAUSE
Let that feeling of relaxation travel down from your shoulders right down your back

LONG PAUSE
Right down your right leg, down through the muscles, through your knee, down through the ankle

PAUSE
To your foot, right down to your toes

LONG PAUSE
Let the feeling of relaxation now travel down your left leg

PAUSE
Down through the muscles, down through your knee, down through your ankle

PAUSE
To your foot, right down to your toes

LONG PAUSE
I'll give you a few moments now

PAUSE
To allow you to concentrate on any part of your body that you would like to relax even further

15-SECOND PAUSE MINIMUM
I want you to concentrate on your breathing again

PAUSE
Notice as you breathe

PAUSE
On each out-breath you feel more relaxed

LONG PAUSE
I would like you in your mind to say the number 'one'

PAUSE (NB. Option: if the number 'one' evokes an emotion then participants are asked to choose another number of their choice)

And say it every time you breathe out

LONG PAUSE
This will help you to push away any unwanted thoughts you may have

PAUSE
Each time you breathe out just say the number in your mind

30-SECOND PAUSE (NB. Option: Up to 20 minutes pause here if an extended session is required. If extended then regular input from the therapist or trainer is needed to remind the participants to repeat the mantra 'one' or whatever number they have chosen)

I want you now

PAUSE
To think of your favourite relaxing place

PAUSE
I want you to concentrate

PAUSE
On your favourite relaxing place

LONG PAUSE
Try and see it in your mind's eye

LONG PAUSE
Look at the colours

PAUSE
Perhaps concentrate on one of the colours now

PAUSE
Maybe one of your favourite colours if it's there

LONG PAUSE
Now concentrate on any sounds or noises in your favourite relaxing place

LONG PAUSE
Now concentrate on any smells or aromas in your favourite

PAUSE
Relaxing place

LONG PAUSE
Now just imagine touching something

PAUSE
In your favourite relaxing place

LONG PAUSE
Just imagine how it feels

LONG PAUSE
I want you now to concentrate on your breathing again

PAUSE
Notice once again that every time you breathe out

PAUSE
You feel more

PAUSE
And more relaxed

LONG PAUSE

Whenever you want to in the future you will be able to remember your favourite relaxing place or the breathing exercise and it will help you to relax quickly

LONG PAUSE

In a few moments' time, but not quite yet, I'm going to count three

PAUSE

And you will be able to open your eyes in your own time

PAUSE (Option: go off to sleep if you so wish)

One

PAUSE

Two

PAUSE

Three

PAUSE

Open your eyes in your own time

Key: PAUSE is about 1–3 seconds in duration

LONG PAUSE is about 5–15 seconds in duration

NB. The durations may vary depending upon the time allocated to the relaxation exercise.

Biofeedback. Biofeedback may be used in conjunction with relaxation techniques to indicate the degree of relaxation a client has achieved. One type of instrument in current use measures skin conductivity. If the client feels stressed in some way, his autonomic nervous system is aroused and his skin conductivity increases. The instrument measures GSR (Galvanic Skin Response) and can be used to show clients how different bodily states arising from images, sensations and cognitions can trigger a skin response within seconds. Biofeedback is thus a useful aid in teaching relaxation skills.

Meditation and Yoga are two other relaxation techniques which clients can be taught to help them relax their bodies and divert themselves when they feel anxious or are obsessive-compulsive. A modified form of meditation, known as the Benson relaxation response, employs a simple mantra to help clients to ignore distracting or negative thoughts while they relax. Benson claimed that this response resembles transcendental meditation and decreases a variety of stress-related disorders including blood pressure and heart rate.[6] Benson's technique, modified by Palmer and Dryden, is described briefly in Palmer and Dryden:[7]

1. Find a comfortable position and sit quietly.
2. Close your eyes.
3. Relax your muscles, starting at your face and progress down to your toes.
4. Now concentrate on your breathing. Breathe naturally through your nose. In your mind say the number 'one' as you breathe out.
5. Continue this exercise for a further 10–20 minutes.
6. When you finish, keep your eyes closed for a couple of minutes and sit quietly.

There are many books describing Yoga exercises, including deep breathing techniques, which some clients find useful as aids to relaxation. However, before encouraging a client to undertake Yoga, make sure that he or she is not suffering from any medical condition that makes Yoga-type activities dangerous.

What are the benefits of relaxation techniques when used as stress management strategies? They basically work because they involve a great deal of thought distraction. When, for example, a client is using progressive relaxation she is concentrating on relaxing one set of muscles after another and is forced to think so closely about what she is doing to relax that she consequently finds it very difficult to worry or think about anything else.

Thus clients undergoing relaxation procedures may feel better for a time, but because these techniques are palliative, you had better show them that they will unduly stress themselves again, because they have not yet discovered the specific Irrational Beliefs with which they largely create their anxieties.

Use these relaxation techniques at times, but use them in an REBT framework. Explain to your clients that relaxation can help, but by itself seldom leads to profound personality change. Wagenaar and La Forge quote Burish's assertion (1981) that it was doubtful that biofeedback or any relaxation strategy alone has permanent stress-reducing effects, and conclude with the comment by A.A. Lazarus and Mayne: 'Although relaxation remains the only empirically documented anti-stress procedure to date, it will not resolve difficult problems, cure arcane physiological disorders, or supply requisite interpersonal skills.' Also as Ellis and Abrahms pertinently note:[8]

> ... just as aspirin is palliative but often useful, so are various kinds of relaxing and distracting methods. If you can show [clients] how to relax physically or otherwise to distract themselves, they will often be in a much better frame of mind.... If they have overweening basic anxiety, relaxing methods will only work temporarily and had better also be accompanied by some of the other important REBT methods.

Thus, if your clients suffer from sleep problems, for example, and practise one of the relaxing techniques mentioned here, they may be able to get to sleep more easily. At the same time, however, you can show your clients that insomnia isn't *awful* or *horrible* but only highly inconvenient, and that by using the REBT techniques you have taught them, they can give up their anxieties *about* sleeping, and often sleep much better.

Relaxation techniques may be valuable to bring about a variety of biological changes. They may reduce levels of tension which often lead to more dangerous kinds of physiological stress. They also give clients the breathing space they may need to look at and change the chief source of their stress – their Irrational Beliefs and faulty inferences.

Suggestion and positive imagery

You can help clients who hold negative images of themselves by showing them how to replace negative thinking with 'positive thinking' or positive imagery. This technique was first used by Emile Coué and later by Norman Vincent Peale and Maxwell Maltz. These exponents of the power of positive thinking realized that other people's suggestion works largely because clients turn it into autosuggestion and actively believe in the 'truth' of what some persuasive authority has told them.

As history shows, spellbinders can do enormous harm. But considerable clinical and experimental evidence shows that positive thinking often works. People who have been depressed, paralysed and extremely anxious have used it to convince themselves that they can succeed at various tasks and to live more happily despite many difficulties in their lives.

You can, with certain caveats, use suggestion to help a number of clients. Use it, for example, with clients who, for one reason or another, have limited ability to respond to more elegant forms of REBT – such as young children and older, inflexible adults, and clients with severe personality disorders. Recognize, however, that positive thinking has its distinct limitations. As Jerome Frank has argued, conversion lies at the heart of a great deal of what we call psychotherapy.[9] Yes, some of your clients, because of your or their own positive suggestion, may be converted to believing that they *can* succeed, *can* win others' approval and do have intrinsic worth. Such positive thinking can bring excellent results, because these clients change their basic philosophy from 'I *can't* succeed therefore I'm worthless!' to 'I *can* succeed and therefore I'm a worthwhile person!'

Positive thinking and positive imagery, however, have distinct limitations, including:

1. While positively imagining themselves succeeding, your clients may retain their fundamental philosophy that they would be worthless if they failed. They have to *keep* imagining themselves succeeding and being approved by others to remain unanxious about failing.
2. Clients who actually succeed more by using positive thinking may reinforce their Belief, 'I am doing well *therefore* I have worth'. They rarely use it to accept themselves *un*conditionally.
3. Positive thinking often encourages Pollyannaism which leads to disillusionment when your clients' Belief that they unquestionably *will* do well turns out to be false.

Positive suggestion and autosuggestion have a certain power and appeal for clients who resist using elegant REBT. But use these techniques with caution and with full knowledge of their limitations. Your aim in *elegant* REBT is to encourage your clients to become *less* suggestible, to think for themselves, to choose their own lifestyle, rather than to blindly follow your or other persons' agendas and dictates. You had better often employ rational emotive imagery rather than positive thinking and imagery with their intrinsic limitations and dangers.

Hypnosis

As Hippolyte Bernheim and Emile Coué realized, hypnosis largely works through suggestion, and an individual's self-suggestion when she or he accepts the hypnotist's suggestions. Ellis has stated that REBT is closely related to hypnosis. For example, he shows that hypnosis usually consists of giving clients strong, repeated, rational coping statements and inducing clients to act on them, while REBT teaches them to challenge and dispute their own negative self-statements and irrational beliefs.[10] Both systems assume that humans upset themselves with faulty ideas, images and cognitions and that clients can be taught to change their faulty beliefs and assumptions and overcome their disturbed feelings and behaviour.

In addition, hypnosis and REBT are highly active-directive, they emphasize homework assignments and *in vivo* desensitization and urge clients to actively work against their LFT and self-defeating behaviours. Because of this degree of overlap between some of the basic theories and practices of REBT and hypnotherapy, Ellis sometimes combines REBT with hypnosis. Indeed, Ellis notes that when used in conjunction with hypnosis, REBT is effective because clients are shown (a) that they have acquired several irrational ideas; (b) that when they believe these IBs they are almost bound to become emotionally disturbed; and (c) that the way to overcome their disturbance is to see that their ideas are irrational, to challenge and weaken them with counter-suggestion, and to replace them with more rational ideas.

To illustrate the use of the REBT hypnotic procedure we include below a brief description of and excerpts from a hypnotherapy session conducted by Albert Ellis which originally appeared in Ellis's paper 'Anxiety about anxiety'.[11]

Case description

This is the case of a 33-year-old unmarried female borderline personality disorder who had a 20-year history of being severely anxious about her school, work, love and sex performances and who became classically anxious about her anxiety, had a severe case of phrenophobia, and was sure that she would end up without friends, lovers or money. Actually, she was quite attractive, could function quite well sexually when she felt secure with a love partner (which was rare), and made a large salary as a sales manager.

Although this client had received 13 sessions of REBT and had notably decreased her feelings of terror about falling in love, sex and business, she would fall back a few weeks later and make herself exceptionally upset – especially about her anxiety itself. After hearing that one of her friends was helped to stop smoking by hypnotherapy she asked her therapist if he used it along with REBT. The therapist explained that he sometimes did use hypnotherapy but did not encourage clients to resort to it because they thought of it as a form of magic and used it instead of working at REBT.

However, the therapist agreed to try it with her and used it once. The following is a shortened transcript of the first and only session Dr Ellis had with his client. It is preceded by a brief description of the hypnotic procedure used:

THE HYPNOTIC PROCEDURE

First, clients are put into what is usually a light hypnotic (or deeply relaxed) state, using a modified version of Jacobson's (1938) progressive relaxation technique, which takes only about ten minutes to effect. The therapist then follows this with ten minutes of REBT instruction, designed to show clients that they have a few specific Irrational Beliefs (IBs) with which they are creating some major problem (e.g. anxiety, depression, rage or self-downing) and that if they keep actively and strongly disputing these IBs (as the therapist has previously taught them to do in several nonhypnotic sessions), they will change their beliefs – and thereby also appreciably change their self-defeating feelings and behaviours that stem from and reinforce these IBs. As Ellis explains:

> The unique feature of this REBT hypnotic procedure is that I often use it only once, for a single session, to work on a client's main presenting problem. I record both the 10 minutes of hypnotic relaxation induction plus the following ten minutes of REBT instruction on a 60-minute audio cassette. I give the cassette to the clients to keep listening to every day, at least once a day, for the next 30 to 60 days. Using this method, I only see the clients for a single 30-minute hypnotic session; but they get 15, 30, or more hours of recorded REBT hypnotic therapy at their own home or office for the next month or two; and if they actually use this time as I direct them to do, they often develop deeper and deeper trance states, even though during the original live session they develop only a very light trance – or, as many of them report, no real trance state at all.

HYPNOTIC SESSION

As the therapist nears the end of the relaxation induction the client becomes more and more relaxed, listening only to the sound of the therapist's voice, repeating and repeating the same, soothing, relaxing message:

> ... Your eyes are getting heavier and heavier and you want to let yourself sink, you're trying to let yourself sink, into a deeper, deeper, relaxed state.... You're only listening to the sound of my voice, that's all you're focusing on, that's all you want to hear – the sound of my voice. And you're going to do what I tell you to do, because you *want to*, you *want* to do it. You want to stay in this relaxed state and be fully aware of my voice and do what I tell you to do because you *want* to do it, you *want* to be relaxed. You *want* to rid yourself of your anxiety and you *know* that this will help you relax and listen, relax and listen, go into a fully free and relaxed state.

> You're only focusing on my voice and you're going to listen carefully to what I'm telling you. You're going to remember everything I tell you. And after you awake from this relaxed, hypnotic state, you're going to feel very good. Because you're going to remember everything and use what you hear – use it for you. Use it to put away all your anxiety and all your anxiety *about* your anxiety. Whenever you feel anxious about anything, you're going to remember what I'm telling you now, in this relaxed state, and you're going to fully focus on it, concentrate on it very well, and do exactly what we're talking about – relax and get rid of your anxiety, relax and get rid of your anxiety.

At this point the therapist begins to deliver the REBT part of the hypnotic session:

> Whenever you get anxious about anything, you're going to realize that the reason you're anxious is because you're saying to yourself, telling yourself 'I *must* succeed! I *must*

succeed! I *must* do this, or I *must* not do that!' You will clearly see and fully accept that your anxiety comes from your self-statement. It doesn't come from without. It doesn't come from other people. *You* make yourself anxious, by demanding that something *must* go well or *must* not exist. It's *your* demand that makes you anxious. It's always you and your self-talk; and therefore *you* control it and *you* can change it.

You're going to realize 'I make myself anxious. I don't *have* to keep making myself anxious, if I give up my demands, my musts, my shoulds, my oughts. If I really accept what is, accept things the way they are, then I won't be anxious. I can always make myself unanxious by giving up my musts, by relaxing – by wanting and wishing for things, but not *needing*, not *insisting*, not *demanding*, not *musturbating* about them.'

You're going to keep telling yourself 'I can *ask* for things, I can *wish*, but I do not *need* what I want! There is nothing I *must* have; and there is nothing I *must* avoid, including my anxiety. I'd *like* to get rid of this anxiety. I *can* get rid of it. I'm *going* to get rid of it. But if I tell myself "I *must* not be anxious! I *must* not be anxious! I *must* be unanxious!" then I'll be anxious.

'Nothing will kill me. Anxiety won't kill me. Lack of sex won't kill me. There are lots of unpleasant things in the world that I don't like, but I can *stand* them, I don't *have* to get rid of them. If I'm anxious, I'm anxious – too damn bad! Because *I* control my emotional destiny – as long as I feel that I don't *have* to do anything, that I have to succeed at anything. That's what destroys me – the idea that I *have* to be sexy or I have to succeed at sex. Or that I *have* to get rid of my anxiety.' In your regular life, after listening to this tape regularly, you're going to think and to keep thinking these things. Whenever you're anxious, you'll look at what you're doing to *make* yourself anxious, and you'll give up your demands and your musts. You'll dispute your ideas that 'I *must* do well! I *must* get people to like me! They *must* not criticize me! It's terrible when they criticize me!' You'll keep asking yourself 'Why *must* I do well? Why do I *have* to be a great sex partner? It would be *nice* if people liked me, but they don't *have* to. I do not *need* their approval. If they criticize me, if they blame me, or they think I'm too sexy or too little sexy, too damn bad! I do not *need* their approval, I'd *like* it, but I don't *need* it. I'd also *like* to be un-anxious, but there's no reason why I *must* be. Yes, there's no reason why I *must* be. It's just *preferable*. None of these things I fail at are going to kill me.

'And when I die, as I eventually will, so I die! Death is not horrible, it's a state of *no* feeling. It's exactly the same state I was in before I was born. I won't feel *anything*. So I certainly need not be afraid of that! And even if I get very anxious and go crazy, that too isn't terrible. If I tell myself "I *must* not go crazy! I *must* not go crazy!" then I'll make myself crazy! But even if I'm crazy, so I'm crazy! I can *live* with it even if I'm in a mental hospital. I can *live* and not depress myself about it. *Nothing* is terrible – even when people don't like me, even when I'm acting stupidly, even when I'm very anxious! *Nothing* is terrible! I *can* stand it! It's only a pain in the ass!'

Now this is what you're going to think in your everyday life. Whenever you get anxious about anything, you're going to see what you are anxious about, you're going to realize that you are demanding something, saying 'It *must* be so! I *must* get well! I *must* not do the wrong thing! I *must* not be anxious!' And you're going to stop and say 'You know – I don't need that nonsense. If these things happen, they happen. It's not the end of the world! I'd *like* to be unanxious, I'd *like* to get along with people, I'd *like* to have good sex. But if I don't, I *don't! Tough!* It's not the end of everything. I can always be a happy human *in spite* of failures and hassles. If I don't *demand*, if I don't *insist*, if I don't say "I must, I must!" Musts are crazy. My *desires* are all right. But, again, I don't *need* what I *want!*' Now this is what you're going to keep working at in your everyday life.

You're going to keep using your head, your thinking ability, to focus, to concentrate on ridding yourself of your anxiety – just as you're listening and concentrating right now. Your concentration will get better and better. You're going to be more and more in control of your thoughts and your feelings. You will keep realizing that *you* create your anxiety, *you* make yourself upset, and *you* don't have to, you never have to keep doing so. You can always give up your anxiety. You can always change. You can always relax, and relax, and relax, and not take *anyone*, not take *anything* too seriously.

This is what you're going to remember and work at when you get out of this relaxed state. This idea is what you're going to take with you all day, every day. '*I* control me. I don't *have* to upset myself about anything. If I do upset myself, too bad. I may feel upset for a while but it won't ruin my life or kill me. And I can be anxious without putting myself down, without saying "I must not be anxious!" At times I will make myself anxious, but I can give up my anxiety, if I don't *demand* that I be unanxious.'

And you're going to get better and better about thinking in this rational way. You'll become more in control of you. Never *totally* in control, because nobody ever is totally unanxious. But you'll make yourself much less anxious and able to live with it when you are anxious. And if you live with it, it will go away. Nothing is terrible, not even anxiety. That's what you're going to realize and to keep thinking about until you really, really believe it.

Now you feel nice and warm and fully relaxed. In a few minutes I'm going to tell you to come out of this relaxed, hypnotic state. You will then have a good day. You will feel fine when you come out of this state. You will experience no ill effects of the hypnosis. You will remember everything I just said to you and will keep working at using it. And you will play this tape every day for the next 30 days. You will listen to it every day until you really believe it and follow it. Eventually you will be able to follow its directions and to think your way out of anxiety and out of anxiety *about* being anxious without the tape.

You will then be able to release yourself from anxiety by yourself. You can always relax and use the antianxiety technique you will learn by listening to the tape. You can always accept yourself *with* your anxiety and can stop telling yourself 'I *must* not be anxious! I *must* not be anxious!' Just tell yourself 'I don't *like* anxiety, I'll work to give it up. I'll conquer it. I'll control myself, control my own emotional destiny. I can always relax, make myself feel easy and free and nice, just as I feel now, get away from cares for a while and then feel unanxious. But I can more elegantly accept myself first with my anxiety, stop fighting it desperately, and stop telling myself it's awful to be anxious. Then I can go back to the original anxiety and get rid of it by refusing to awfulize about failing and vigorously disputing my Irrational Beliefs, "I must do well! I must not be disapproved!"'

Now you feel good, you feel relaxed, and in a couple of minutes, I'm going to count to three and when I count to three you will awake and feel quite alive, have a good day, and experience no bad effects, no headaches, no physical discomfort! Everything is going to be fine and you'll have a good day. You will remember all this and, as I said, you will listen to this tape whenever you possibly can, at least once a day. And you will think and act more and more on its message. You'll be able to control yourself and reduce your anxiety appreciably. And when you do feel anxious you'll live with the anxiety, accept it, and refuse to panic yourself about it. All right, I'm going to count to three and when I say *three* you'll wake and be fully alive and alert and feel great for the rest of the day. One, two, three!

Therapeutic outcome

Ellis reported the outcome of his session with his client as follows:

My client used the recording of her hypnotic REBT session once or twice a day for the next 45 days and reported a significant decrease in her anxiety level, and especially in her anxiety about her anxiety. She stopped being phrenophobic, convinced herself that if she had a breakdown and went into a mental hospital it would be highly inconvenient but not horrible or shameful, and then hardly thought at all about going crazy. When she did, she was able to feel comfortable within a few minutes by strongly telling herself 'So I'll be crazy! Tough! I'm sure I won't stay that way very long – and if I do, that will just be tougher. But not shameful! No matter how crazy I am, I'll never be a turd for being that way!'

As she began to get over her anxiety about her anxiety, this woman's enormous fears of failure, particularly of sex failure, for a while almost completely disappeared. When, weeks later, they reappeared, they were relatively light, and she was almost invariably able to cope successfully with them. She continued in REBT nonhypnotic treatment for 14 months more, but only had 18 half-hour sessions during that time. For the last eleven years she has maintained her gains, with occasional moderate setbacks when a love affair ended, and is now happily married and unanxiously highly productive. Once in a while she still listens to the original hypnotic tape and believes that it was quite instrumental in helping her make much greater progress than she had previously made in REBT.

I tend to agree with her, partly because I have used similar taped sessions to good avail with about 80 other clients (although with little or no success with 18 others). One important question I have not yet resolved is: Does the benefit presumably derived from this tape of recorded hypnotic sessions stem from the use of the entire 30-minute tape, including the hypnotic relaxation instructions, or would equal benefit stem from the client's listening a number of times to the 10 minutes of REBT instruction on the tape even if this were heard apart from the hypnotic section? I have tried to induce several researchers to do a controlled study of this question but so far no one, to my knowledge, has done so. Until then, I shall continue to use this recorded hypnosis-REBT procedure with some amount of faith in the clinical results I have thus far achieved with it.

Practitioners wishing to obtain information on how to use relaxation and hypnosis in stress management should consult Stephen Palmer's booklet *Multimodal Techniques:*

Relaxation and Hypnosis, which contains a wealth of practical detail and can also be used with stress counselling and psychotherapy clients.[12]

Ellis found that the depth of the trance achieved by his clients did not seem to make much difference because, when he gave them posthypnotic suggestions to work at using REBT in their regular lives, clients usually carried out his suggestions regardless of whether they achieved any deep trance state.[13]

Limitations of hypnosis

Because one of the main purposes of REBT is to help clients effect a profound, *highly conscious* philosophic change it differs from most other hypnotic therapies in its view that the process of clients making the transition from their old irrational thinking and dysfunctional behaviours to more rational views and productive behaviours involves their using a very wide awake, deliberately conscious programme of cognitive, emotive and behavioural re-conditioning. Ellis therefore prefers to first use regular REBT without hypnosis, and then, if that does not work, to use hypnosis with REBT. Briefly, he uses hypnosis mainly in special instances because REBT espouses helping people to think for themselves, to be *less* suggestible, and not to unthinkingly adopt suggestions from a hypnotist or anyone else.[14]

REBT shows clients how they can be independent of their therapists, stand on their own feet, and construct ways of helping themselves to cope when they feel stressed at various times throughout their lives. By contrast, some forms of hypnosis imply that they need an authoritative person for support.

In spite of the above disadvantages, hypnosis combined with REBT can be used with clients who ask for it. Its main advantage is that since these clients believe in the magic of hypnosis, they are more likely to work at using REBT when it is combined with hypnotism. As we saw, when Ellis does hypnotherapy with REBT, the sessions are tape-recorded and the clients take these tapes home with them and listen to them 20 to 30 times. As they do so, the frequent repetition of the REBT messages on the tape gets through to them, making it more likely that the clients will respond to the rational self-statements on the tape and keep doing their homework. Hypnosis is by no means an elegant therapy, but when combined with REBT it can significantly help clients who resist using REBT's cognitive, emotive and behavioural methods to become less distressed about the stressors in their lives.

Interpretation of defences

Humans often tend to become defensive when confronted with their failings. Instead of honestly admitting their shortcomings, they practise various covering up strategies such as rationalization, avoidance, denial and projecting blame on to others. Because these defensive tactics block them from tackling and ridding themselves of some of their most troubling problems, REBT practitioners look for evidence of defensiveness and deal with it first, so that clients are more likely to bring out the problem(s) they may be loath to mention.

Rational emotive behaviour theory assumes that defences largely stem from self-condemnation. So you had better identify and dispute the Irrational Beliefs that underlie your clients' self-condemnation and help them to replace these ideas with those leading to unconditional self-acceptance (USA).

When you deal with defensive clients, disclose their cavilling and show them that no matter what 'stupid', 'shameful' or antisocial act they performed, they are not bad persons. As you demonstrate that you fully accept *them* and teach them how to achieve self-acceptance you can then collaborate with them to work at minimizing their poor behaviours.

It is important to realize that accepting a person who has committed a misdeed does not mean that you accept that person's act. Let's take a fairly common example. Sharon comes to you for help to stop feeling guilty – that is, self-castigating – about having slept with her best friend's husband. You succeed in helping Sharon to overcome her feeling of guilt and to feel only remorse over betraying her best friend's trust. This does not mean that you give Sharon an excuse for continuing to act immorally. Quite the opposite! You help her see that her behaviour was still immoral. The rational alternative to guilt is remorse. This is based on the Rational Belief 'I wish I hadn't broken my moral code by betraying my best friend behind her back, but there is no reason why I *absolutely should not* have broken it. I broke it because of the thoughts that were going through my head at the time. Now let me accept myself and learn from my unethical behaviour so that I can act better in future.'

Dryden describes the situation thus: The principle of emotional responsibility, a central tenet of REBT,

> ... encourages the person to take responsibility for her actions and for her disturbed (guilt) feelings. It further encourages the person to challenge her irrational, guilt-producing beliefs, and adopt a rational remorse-invoking philosophy so that she can learn from her past behaviour, make appropriate amends and take responsibility for her future behaviour.

In other words, remorse does not provide the person with a 'cop-out' or excuse for continuing to act immorally. Self-responsibility for one's own behaviour has always been emphasized throughout REBT theory and practice.[15]

Reattribution therapy

People easily tend to attribute motives and intentions to others that are often wide of the mark and thereby often needlessly disturb themselves. Paranoid individuals in particular easily convince themselves that the world is against them and that they can't trust anybody.

Whenever your clients complain that someone is deliberately acting unfairly or nastily towards them and is deliberately trying to do them in, check their attributions. Are other explanations possible? Encourage your client to check out their inferences and to look for alternative explanations. False attributions spring from faulty inferences. So try to uncover the automatic thoughts or inferences that lead to your clients' disturbance and encourage them to question and challenge these surmises. Once they change their faulty inferences and attributions, you can encourage them to proceed to identify and dispute the core Irrational Beliefs underlying their faulty inferences and misattributions such as 'Because James *absolutely has to be* 100 per cent on my side, and he seems to favour me less than that, I am sure he hates me and is plotting against me!'

Usually, you prefer to get to clients' core IBs directly and to challenge them as quickly as possible, rather than focus on their inferences. However, if a client presents a problem that appears to be linked to faulty attributions, you may choose first to help her to challenge the validity of her inferences and to give up her semi-paranoid attributions, but don't stop there! Also encourage your client to identify and dispute the core IBs that underlie her attributions, so that she becomes better able to tackle her practical life problems.

Skill training

REBT helps people acquire a humanistic, existential, self-actualizing and socially oriented philosophy, but it also is highly practical and behavioural. It encourages clients to philosophically push themselves to acquire useful skills; but it also shows that social skill training – such as communication and assertion training – help people to change their thinking and make themselves less prone to emotional distress. So to do stress inoculation, you had better be ready to do some effective skill training with your clients.[16]

Skill training has a number of advantages, because it shows clients that they can make 'impossible' changes; that they can change some of their rigid thinking and disturbed feelings by *acting* against them; and that they can achieve more social, sexual, vocational and other success and pleasure. When done by itself, with little cognitive restructuring, skill training also has distinct limitations. It can encourage clients to foolishly esteem their *self* rather than their improved performances. It motivates some clients to quit therapy too early, after they have gained some skills but *not* surrendered their Irrational Beliefs. It doesn't work well unless clients first acquire higher frustration tolerance, so that they work hard to acquire important skills and also keep working and using them in order to maintain them. People who are still basically disturbed can use their skills badly, antisocially, to gain short-range instead of long-range satisfactions, and to louse themselves up in spite of their proficiencies. Look, for instance, at the many talented artists, scientists, entertainers and business tycoons whose efficacy hardly stopped them from leading highly panicked and depressed lives!

By all means, then, use skill training selectively – and encourage your clients to do likewise. They had better *think* carefully about what kind of skills would be *individually* best for them – and not for 'everyone' or for the 'average' person – as I (A.E.) pointed out almost 20 years ago.

In an even broader sense, skill training in the field of counselling had better include teaching clients the more complex cognitive skills of viewing their fundamental goals and values, clarifying and assessing the ramifications of these values, noting the practical results (both beneficial and pernicious) to which they lead, at times wilfully and intentionally changing these goals and values, and constantly reconsidering and modifying the specific skills and the specific skill training methods that seem to promote human health and happiness.[17]

We believe that this kind of cognitively arrived at and constantly appraised and revised skill training will render this highly effective counselling method even more useful to a wide range of clients, and hopefully minimize some of the limitations and dangers of some present-day skill training.

Ending counselling

The time to consider ending rational emotive behaviour counselling arises when you have evidence that your clients have successfully overcome the problems that brought them to counselling and have shown that they can use REBT methods to deal with anticipated future problems. Preferably, you are then teaching them to become their own counsellor today and tomorrow.

If some of your clients express doubts about their ability to cope on their own after counselling has ended, ask for an example of a problem or situation they think they cannot cope with on their own. Dryden offers the useful suggestion that you give your clients a problem situation they think they cannot cope with as a home-work assignment. A few follow-up sessions can be negotiated to enable you to monitor their progress.

There is no absolute or final end to the REBT counselling process because, as Dryden notes, '... in most cases you would probably want your client to contact you for further help if they have struggled on their own for a reasonably long time to put into practice the rational emotive behaviour problem-solving method without success'.[18]

NOTES

1. Dryden, 1995a; Ellis, 1994a, 1995c.
2. Ellis, 1978, p. 125.
3. Wolpe and Lazarus, 1966.
4. Palmer and Dryden, 1995, p. 132.
5. Palmer, 1993d, pp. 17–23.
6. Benson, 1975.
7. Palmer and Dryden, 1995, p. 139.
8. Burish, 1981; Ellis and Abrahms, 1978, Lazarus and Mayne, 1990.
9. Frank, 1973.
10. Ellis, 1986, 1993d.
11. Ellis, 1986.
12. Palmer, 1993d.
13. Ellis, 1986, 1993d.
14. Ellis, 1993d, 1995c.
15. Dryden, 1995a, p. 440.
16. Ellis, 1977f, 1996.
17. Ellis, 1977f.
18. Dryden, 1990b.

CHAPTER 7

Brief Psychotherapy and Crisis Intervention in Rational Emotive Behaviour Therapy

People who undergo some unusual, unexpected and highly stressful experience, such as the breakup of a relationship that occurs suddenly, like a bolt from the blue, may require brief crisis intervention. REBT is well suited for brief crisis intervention because, as Ellis has noted, REBT is intrinsically brief.[1]

Indications for brief REBT

At the beginning of therapy, it is important to assess your client's suitability for brief REBT. This comes down to making a judgement as to whether or not your client is functioning sufficiently well in life to respond constructively to brief REBT. You will find a comprehensive discussion of the pros and cons of offering brief REBT to clients in Dryden's book *Brief Rational Emotive Behaviour Therapy*.[2] Here, we note some of the more salient points.

1. First, you had better carry out, or arrange for someone else to carry out, a thorough formal assessment of your potential client's level of psychological functioning. You may, for example, arrange with a psychiatrist to carry out a full mental status examination and full personal history to help you decide whether or not this particular individual is likely to be a good candidate for brief REBT.
2. You may wish to form an opinion of your client's ability to understand the basic goals of effective REBT and her willingness and ability to accept and carry out her responsibilities in the task domain.
3. A helpful indication of future progress is whether or not you and your client are developing a good working bond early in the counselling relationship. If your client openly discusses her problems with you and a good rapport is developing between you, the indications for brief REBT are favourable.
4. Provided your client's physical well-being is not a problem you may proceed as quickly as is feasible with the process of cognitively restructuring the core Irrational Beliefs that underpin your client's psychological disturbances. In addition to the cognitive, emotive-evocative and behavioural methods outlined in previous

chapters, you may find useful suggestions for crisis intervention approaches in R.E. McMullin's *Handbook of Cognitive Therapy Techniques* (pp. 269–71).[3]

Contraindications for brief therapy

Before deciding to offer brief REBT as a response to a client's crisis situation, several contraindications had better be taken into account. These are:

1. If, for example, in the first session the person seems reticent to 'open up', or appears to be antipathetic to you or your counselling style, the chances are this person is not a good candidate for brief REBT, at least with you as her therapist. In this case, a suitable referral may be advisable.
2. The person doesn't accept the REBT view of psychological disturbance and its treatment.
3. The person does not accept that she will find helpful the therapeutic tasks that REBT requires of therapist and client.
4. The person is disinclined or unable to carry out homework assignments.
5. The person has a long history of psychological disturbance that still appears to be present.

As Dryden observes,

> Between the definite indications and contraindications for brief REBT lies the grey area where a person may meet some of the indications for brief REBT, but not others. As long as the person does not meet any of the contraindications listed above, the only guidance I can give is that the greater the number of indications present, the more likely it is that the person is suitable for brief REBT. It is useful to discuss cases that fall into the grey area with your supervisor.[4]

In general, once you are proceeding with brief REBT, monitor your client's response to treatment and be prepared to 'change tack' and to modify your treatment plan as necessary. A client may meet all your suitability criteria for brief REBT, but still fail to respond productively. If this occurs, you may refer your client to another therapist, enlist some specialist help, or suggest a period of slower-paced longer-term counselling. Ellis's book *Better, Deeper and More Enduring Brief Therapy* provides an excellent coverage of the subject.[5]

Case illustration

Tina, a 35-year-old single woman of Afro-European descent and the mother of three young children, had been brought to hospital in an unconscious state following an emergency telephone call from her mother who had found her daughter lying at home, apparently in a coma. Tina's boyfriend, who had been living with her at that time, had suddenly left her. She phoned her mother sounding hysterical, to report that her boyfriend had not only left her, but had ransacked Tina's house, taking with him everything of value that Tina possessed, and leaving Tina with nothing but her personal clothing. He also took some £50 in cash and notes that Tina had kept for use in an emergency in a drawer in her bedroom. A scribbled note warned her against following him or taking any action to recover her stolen property. As she sobbed out her story to her mother, Tina suddenly exclaimed 'After what's happened to me I'd be better off dead!'

Fearing for her daughter's safety, Tina's mother hurried over to Tina's house and found Tina lying on the sofa unconscious, with her three young children wandering around the house crying and obviously in a very distressed state. An emergency call for an ambulance brought a quick response. Tina was rushed to hospital while her mother took Tina's three children home with her, to temporarily look after them.

At the hospital, tests revealed that Tina had swallowed a heavy, but not lethal, dose of Valium. Based upon the information supplied by Tina's mother, the medical staff concluded that Tina's drug overdose was an impulsive attempt to escape the pain of loss and betrayal by her boyfriend, rather than a real attempt at suicide.

Once Tina had recovered from the physical effects of her overdose of Valium, a mental status examination revealed no obvious mental disorder. She was not hallucinating, and although at times she sounded very agitated, and at other times somewhat depressed, she seemed to be reasonably well oriented. She had no family history of mental disorder, and in spite of her pattern of unstable relationships and her bearing three children from different partners, there seemed no good reason to keep her in hospital. Also, as she continually sought assurance that her children were being properly looked after, it was decided to allow her to return home.

She was prescribed a tri-cyclic anti-depressant before being discharged from hospital, but because she was still very disturbed, her attending psychiatrist recommended out-patient intensive psychotherapy as soon as possible. He also suggested her stress reduction programme should include relaxation training, development of coping skills and advice on nutrition. Arrangements were then made for Tina to see a rational emotive behaviour therapist.

In a crisis situation like this one, your main objective may well be to help the client through the crisis stage of her life as soon as possible. Symptom removal, while not ideal therapy, may therefore be your main goal at this stage. Later, after the client has been helped to get over the crisis situation, and is functioning much better, you may encourage her to work towards more elegant basic personality change.

THE FIRST SESSION

As Tina described what had happened in her relationship with her boyfriend, the therapist listened and empathized with her shocking experience of rejection and betrayal of trust. 'How could he do this to me, after telling me he loved me and after all I did for him?' Tina would ask repeatedly. And the answer, as we all know, is 'Easily'. However, at this stage, the therapist concentrated on empathizing with Tina and showing her by his attitude that he unconditionally accepted her and that her own severe reactions to her traumatic experiences were expectable and fairly common. He stressed that in no way would it help Tina to blame herself for her lover's actions. Once she saw that the therapist accepted her and viewed her distressed symptoms as expectable rather than as abnormal or indicative of a mental breakdown, Tina felt reassured that she wasn't going crazy and she began to listen to the therapist as he began to explain the ABC model of emotional disturbance.

TINA'S ABC

First, the therapist decided to find out what had triggered Tina's breakdown. What helped Tina see A, her traumatic experience, as so devastating?

Tina: When I first met my boyfriend, he seemed very nice. He told me he had a good job, and eventually he promised to look after me. My two older children were at nursery and junior school during the day, and my youngest child stayed at home with me.

Therapist: So you weren't going out to work at that time?

Tina: No. Anyway, I eventually invited him to move in with me, after he had said he would help out with the finances.

Therapist: What work did your boyfriend actually do?

Tina: Well, I was never very sure. I think I know now what he was up to, but at the time he just said he travelled a bit and sold things. He was very vague about what he actually did, and he gave me the impression that it was really none of my business. Then, one day he suggested I get myself a job, because, he said he hadn't been doing so well lately, and that we needed more money. So I got this job I have now in the women's clothing store and I arranged for a professional child minder to look after my youngest child until I got home from work.

Therapist: And then what happened?

Tina: Well, he seemed to be spending more time at home just sitting around and not doing very much. It was then that I asked him what he actually did to earn money, and he got very angry and told me to forget it, that it was his own business, and it didn't concern me. He even told me that if I persisted in asking him questions about what he did, he would leave me. But I didn't believe him. Here he was, enjoying the comforts of my house, while I'm out at work, so he was having it pretty good, I thought, and not likely to give it all up.

Therapist: I see. So, what brought about the breakup?

Tina: One night I got home a little earlier than usual. When I came into the room, there he was sitting with a few of his pals and there was a smell in the room of smoke, which seemed to me like cannabis. After they'd gone, I asked him what he'd been smoking, and he said 'Oh, it was nothing, forget it'. Well, I wasn't going to have that, especially with young children in the house. So later on that evening, I said to him 'You were all smoking cannabis just before I got home, weren't you?' And he said 'Well, so what?' So then I said 'You're into drugs, aren't you? That's how you make your money, pushing drugs, isn't it?' Then he went into a terrible rage and shouted, as he slammed out of the house, that he was never coming back. But I still didn't believe him. He'd threatened before to leave me and he hadn't.

Therapist: What happened next?

Tina: Well he didn't come home that night, and in the morning I went to work as usual. It was when I came home that evening that I saw what had happened. He had driven back to the house during the day when I was out at work, he had a key, you see, and well, you know what happened. I never thought he could do such a thing! He took everything of value I had. That was his way of punishing me, I suppose. And that note he left, threatening to come back and harm me if I reported him to the police or even tried to follow him – how could he do such a thing to somebody he said he loved?

Therapist: People do all sorts of things, Tina – nasty, cruel, stupid things – because that is the way they are, fallible, screwed up humans. But let's look now at what you felt about the way you were treated.

Tina: I felt awful, absolutely devastated. It was bad enough being walked out on – and that was the fourth time it's happened to me, you know – four times some so-and-so of a man has enjoyed bed and board at my expense and then walked out on me. And now this! I just can't take any more!

At this point, Tina began to sob quietly. After a few minutes, she dried her eyes and seemed more composed.

Tina: I'm sorry.

Therapist: There's no need to apologize, Tina. It's perfectly normal to feel extremely sad and sorrowful after what you have experienced. Practically any woman would feel very sorrowful if they'd been treated as you were. We can't go back and change what has happened to you; the past is past. But what we can do is to try to get you to take a different view of what happened to you, so that you begin to *feel* differently about this very bad experience you've had. When you feel differently, you'll have a better chance of functioning better in your daily life. You'll manage to cope better with the problems of bringing up three children, holding a job, looking after your home and managing your life in a less stressful manner, with or without a man to live with. If you want to, you can change the way you are running your life. Are you willing to try?

Tina: Well it would sure be an improvement on what I've put up with over the past few years! I haven't been doing too well lately, have I?

Therapist: No. But if you seriously desire to change some things in your life, you can. I can help you to do that if you are willing to work at it.

Tina: Right, I'm ready to start.

Therapist: OK. You came home and found your boyfriend had gone, and that he had gone through your personal possessions and taken everything you valued. This happened after you discovered he had lied to you about his job, and had tried to conceal the fact that he made his money from selling drugs. He definitely treated you unfairly and immorally. Practically everyone would agree on that. We call that the Activating Event, point A, in our famous ABC theory of emotional disturbance. This ABC theory enables us to explain what actually causes people to feel emotionally devastated when some sudden, totally unexpected and particularly unpleasant event, such as rejection or betrayal, happens to them at point A. The emotional Consequences that follow from A, but are not directly caused by A, we call point C. In your case, the feelings you experienced at C were hurt, anger, horror, despair and disillusionment.

Tina: Yes, but in my case, I know what caused me to feel the bottom had fallen out of my life. He walked out on me and left me with nothing. *That* was what made me feel so awful.

Therapist: Well, it certainly looks like that to you, and probably would look the same to most other people as well. Something very bad happens to you and you feel awful as a result. So you conclude that A, the unpleasant thing that happened to you, caused you to feel shocked, dismayed and horrified. Now let me explain to you in more detail how we humans disturb ourselves – what we think and do to make ourselves panicked, miserable, angry and depressed *about* the unpleasant, painful, negative things that happen to us in life.

At this point, the therapist used the Money Example (see Chapter 4) to explain to Tina that the same event can trigger different feelings in a person, depending on the way they think about it. An alternative to the Money Example, which some clients might relate to better, is the Deserted Island technique, described in detail in Palmer and Dryden's *Counselling for Stress Problems*.[6]

Tina understood the point her therapist made through the Money Example, but still had difficulty in accepting that *it*, the breakup and betrayal, was not the direct cause of her disturbed feelings. People tend to view breakups and betrayals as exceptionally severe stressors which they take more seriously than other kinds of negative life experiences. The suddenness and stark impact of such stressors in people's lives often precipitate severe psychological reactions which, in turn, may lead to dire consequences such as attempted suicide, homicide and acts of violence against property.

You may therefore find it wise to spend a good deal of time in showing your clients that although exceptionally unpleasant events or stressors certainly *contribute* to their disturbances, and may *seem* to directly cause them, they themselves largely create their dysfunctional reactions by holding specific strong Irrational Beliefs, or core dysfunctional philosophies. Not until your clients accept that they probably constructed their own irrational shoulds, oughts and musts, and that only by vigorously and persistently working and practising at thinking, feeling and acting against these IBs will they change them and alleviate their symptoms. Helping your traumatized clients to achieve these insights is your primary therapeutic task. Once that is accomplished, you can then proceed to teach them coping skills to enable them to manage their lives more effectively.

> *Therapist:* Now, Tina, let's see where we're at. Point A stands for the shocking realization that your boyfriend has left you and robbed you of your most valued possessions. C stands for what you felt about it – the feelings of horror, shock, hurt and anger. Now let's look at what you were telling yourself at point B about this very obnoxious experience at A. We are going to do this because your Bs, your Beliefs, your thoughts and ideas about the A situation strongly influence the kind of feelings you have about it.

To help Tina understand this important point, the therapist drew the ABC model on a whiteboard. Underneath each letter he wrote a description of what it stood for. He then checked to see if Tina understood his drawing of the model.

> *Therapist:* Are you with me so far?
> *Tina:* Yes. My thoughts about some happening influence the way I am likely to feel about it. Is that right?
> *Therapist:* Yes. Your thoughts, or the ways you evaluate what has happened to you,

strongly influence how you subsequently feel about it, and also how you subsequently act in relation to what has happened.

Tina: Yes, I remember you saying that A does not cause C. It's B – what goes on in my head that largely determines how I feel.

Therapist: Right. Now let's see what your B consisted of at the moment you discovered your boyfriend had taken everything he wanted from you and left. B consists of two distinct and widely separated Beliefs. The first is a Rational Belief (RB), which was probably something like this: 'What a shock this is! I trusted this man, gave him the run of my house, and now he treats me like this. How unfortunate that I have been subjected to this kind of unfair treatment! I hate the way I have been treated and I hope it never happens again. I'd better see what I can do to stay away from males who seem only to be out for what they can get from me, and to do my best to prevent damage to my family's circumstances in future!' Can you tell me why these Beliefs are rational, Tina?

Tina: I guess it's because they describe what happened to me. They tell it like it is.

Therapist: Right. Your rational statements to yourself about the dismal circumstances you found yourself in at A, can be backed up by pointing to the facts. You suffered a loss, you have been deprived and inconvenienced by what happened to you. Your rational statements or Beliefs acknowledge the badness of the situation. They neither play it down, nor exaggerate it. Also, they show a sensible determination to take whatever steps are necessary to avoid similar unfortunate episodes in future.

Now, if you held only these Rational Beliefs about your betrayal and rejection you would tend to feel very sorry and sad and really annoyed and displeased. These are healthy negative feelings in response to your betrayal by your boyfriend. Furthermore, you would realize that your children, not just you, would suffer as a result of what's happened. You and they would be deprived as you face up to the frustration you are likely to experience as you work to get your life and savings together again. You would see what happened to you as very sad, rather than a holy horror, and your determination to let nothing like it happen again would be a *healthy* response to your misfortune, and it would follow from holding these Rational Beliefs (RBs) about it. The reason why the emotional reactions of annoyance, displeasure, intense sorrow or regret, and sadness, including extreme sadness, are deemed healthy, is because they help you act constructively when faced by unpleasant Activating Events and they lead to your greater enjoyment of life in the longer term.

Tina: Yes, but that wasn't what I really felt at the time. I was totally devastated by it.

Therapist: No, not devastated by *it*, the breakup and betrayal, although that certainly contributed to it. Had the breakup not happened, you would not have felt so disturbed. No, your shock and horror at what had happened and your resort to Valium to put you into a state of oblivion was largely caused by your *Irrational Beliefs* about the breakup and betrayal.

Tina: My Irrational Beliefs?

Therapist: Yes. Your severe symptoms of emotional breakdown didn't come from those Rational Beliefs I've just mentioned, but from a number of specific *Irrational* Beliefs which you strongly held. These were probably along the lines of: 'This *absolutely must* not have happened to me! It is *awful* that I got betrayed by this man! I *can't stand* being treated in this fashion! Since this is the fourth time I've been abandoned by the men in my life, that proves I'm a *weak and inadequate* person who will *never* make it with a good man in any future relationship.'

With these Irrational Beliefs, you could hardly feel anything other than horrified, despairing, self-pitying and self-downing. Then to blot out the pain, you reach for the sleeping pills.

Tina: I just felt 'What's the use of carrying on? I do my best for him and he treats me like dirt.' Later, when I woke up I felt so angry and hurt at the way he'd treated me, especially after all I did for him.

Therapist: Well, your anger and your hurt, as was the case with those other unhealthy emotions you experienced, was sparked by another Irrational Belief.

Tina: Well, you've been right so far, but I find it hard to swallow that I made myself angry because of a belief. It seems more logical to believe that that stinker of a boyfriend made me angry because of that rotten thing he did to me.

Therapist: Yes, I understand how you feel. But I'm going to show you how you can choose to view this very distasteful experience in a very different way than you, and probably most other women in your position, usually view it. It isn't easy to make a fundamental switch in the way you look at life, but if you are willing to make the effort, I believe you will soon see the benefit from it. So let's look at what you were telling yourself to create your anger and hurt at your boyfriend's betrayal.

Your feelings of angry hurt spring from the Irrational Belief 'He *absolutely should not* have treated me in this unfair manner. And because he did treat me in that manner, he is a *rotten person*!' With these thoughts you feel hurt and angry.

Tina: Right, that's exactly what I do feel about him, but what do I do to change the way I view this situation I'm in now? And in what way would that help me?

At this point, the therapist gave Tina a fairly lengthy explanation, flavoured with occasional dashes of humour, concerning why an Irrational Belief is self-defeating, and why a Rational Belief is more productive. Some of his explanation repeated points he had made before, but which he considered needed additional emphasis. Continuing in a very active-directive teaching mode, the therapist explained to Tina why it was essential to identify and Dispute her Irrational Beliefs and to replace these with Rational alternative Beliefs if she wanted to overcome her distress over her betrayal, and to increase her ability to cope more effectively with negative life events in future.

Therapist: I explained to you earlier why the Beliefs you held about your boyfriend's betrayal led to your emotional breakdown, and why they were self-defeating, and therefore irrational. Now let's take your Irrational Beliefs about your boyfriend's betrayal one at a time, using the sensible method of questioning them, that I explained we use, see if you can convince yourself that these IBs make no sense whatever, and can only lead to poor results if you continue to believe them.

Tina: All right, let's begin, but I still think that I didn't deserve to be treated in the way I was treated.

Therapist: OK, we'll look at this issue of deservingness later, if you want. Right now, let's examine those IBs that mainly caused your emotional upheaval following your boyfriend's betrayal.

Tina: OK.

Therapist: Why *must* your boyfriend not have betrayed you?

Tina: Because it was so unfair!

Therapist: Yes, we agree on that. He treated you unfairly. But why *must* he not be unfair to you? Not why is it undesirable that he treated you unfairly. We agree on that. But why *must* he not act unfairly?

Tina: I didn't want him to treat me unfairly and I didn't deserve to be!

Therapist: Maybe so, but does it logically follow that because you demand that you must not be treated unfairly, that therefore your demand *must* be met? Does it logically follow that you *must* get what you think you deserve, and not get what you think you don't deserve? In other words, does it logically follow that whatever you want must be granted?

Tina: No. It doesn't logically follow that because I want something, therefore I must get it.

Therapist: Right. Now ask yourself if your belief is consistent with reality. If you believe that something *absolutely must*, or *must not* occur, it implies that there is some law to that effect, does it not?

Tina: I suppose so.

Therapist: So, do you believe that the world *absolutely must* accede to your demand that you be treated fairly, or at least, not unfairly at all times, with no exception?

Tina: No. I can see that this belief makes no sense. It's unrealistic. If there was some law that I must not be treated unfairly, then I wouldn't be. I'd have no option!

Therapist: Quite so. And the fact is, you *were* treated unfairly – which negates your absolute demand that you mustn't be. Reality is the way it is, no matter how unpleasant or unfair you find it to be.

Tina: Yes, I never thought of it that way, but what you say makes sense now that I do think about it. Things are as they are, and not liking the way they are isn't going to make any difference to their being the way they are.

Therapist: Good. You've acquired a useful insight there. There are very probably no absolute musts, shoulds or oughts in the world. We make them up in our heads. Now let's take a close look at those other Irrational Beliefs or statements you were telling yourself about your betrayal.

Here you are telling yourself 'It is *awful* that I got betrayed by this man, and *I can't stand* being treated in this fashion!' Can you prove that it's awful, not that it's undesirable, but awful – meaning that it is 100 per cent bad? Or even that it is *more* than 100 per cent bad? Badder than it *must* be? For that is what 'awful' really means – so bad that it is totally bad – or right off the scale of badness. Can anything be totally bad – or more than 100 per cent bad?

Tina: Well, it felt pretty bad to me.

Therapist: Yes, we're not saying it isn't bad, or even very bad that you were treated in the way you were treated. I'm asking you, was it as bad as it possibly could be? Was it 101 per cent bad? For that is what awful really means – totally bad, badder than it must be, and even 101 per cent bad.

Tina: Well, no, it wasn't that bad, I admit.

Therapist: Right. In reality anything bad can only lie within a 0–99.999 scale of badness. A helpful way to look at bad events is to put them in their rightful, non-exaggerated context. You can do this by making a comparison of a bad event (such as your ex-boyfriend's betrayal) with other bad events using a scale of badness.

Perhaps it'll make it easier to understand if I illustrate what I mean on a whiteboard.

The therapist then drew Figure 7.1 on a whiteboard.

Scale of badness	100%	Being slowly tortured
	75%	Being seriously injured in a bomb attack
	50%	Having your home burnt down
	25%	Being burgled Failing your exams
	0%	

Figure 7.1

On this scale where does being betrayed and robbed belong? It is certainly bad, but by no means is it comparable in badness to having your home destroyed or being permanently maimed in a bomb attack. Hopefully, this will help you see your misfortunes in perspective, neither playing them down nor exaggerating them.

Your experience was certainly bad, very unfortunate, but it could have been worse. For example, your boyfriend could have destroyed virtually all your property before he left. He could even have set your house on fire! People who are really off the wall can do all manner of stupid, dangerous and destructive acts.

Depending on the time available in the session a more Socratic approach may be used in which clients are asked to recalibrate how bad their unfortunate experience really was. When this is done carefully clients realize that their unfortunate experience was certainly bad, but not 'awful' or 'unbearable' or totally bad as they originally thought.

Tina: Yes, I see that what happened could have been worse. He acted the way he did because he was mad at me.

Therapist: Right. He acted badly, he undoubtedly harmed you, not in any physical sense, but he deprived and inconvenienced you by stealing your property. He has made your economic situation more difficult. Then, by upsetting yourself about his actions, you give yourself a needless pain in the gut. You metaphorically beat yourself over the head because *he* acted badly.

Tina: Yeah, I can see now that I blew up the situation, made it seem worse than it really was.

Therapist: That's right. That's what Irrational Beliefs do when you strongly believe them. They exaggerate the significance of obnoxious events such as your boyfriend's betrayal. That's where your 'terrible', 'awful' feelings come from – your exaggerated, unrealistic evaluations of the negative events you experience in life. You can't avoid life's hassles and various kinds of unfortunate events, but you can refuse to unduly upset yourself about them.

Tina: Yes, and I suppose that it is equally irrational to say 'I can't stand something bad that happens to me'.

Therapist: Right. You obviously can, and did, stand what you believed you couldn't stand, so it makes no sense for anyone to claim they *can't stand* what they don't *like*. If you really couldn't stand being betrayed by your boyfriend, or any other misfortune that might hit you for that matter, you would literally come apart at the seams!

Tina: (laughing): Well, I'm still in one piece, at least!

Therapist: Yes, the fact is that you *can* stand virtually anything until you die.

Tina: I never thought of that before, but it makes sense.

Therapist: Right. Now, let's take your other IB about yourself: 'I'm a *weak* and *inadequate* person who will *never* make it with a good man in any future relationship.' Can you rationally support that belief?

Tina: Well, that's how it looks to me right now.

Therapist: That's how you *define* it right now. But prove to me that you are a weak, inadequate person who will never make it with a good man in future.

Tina: I've screwed up so many times already by getting involved with the wrong kind of guys.

Therapist: That only proves that *so far* you have picked the wrong men, or done foolish things, with them. You still have not shown me why you can *never* have a good relationship with the kind of compatible person who might be right for you in the kind of committed, long-term relationship you told me you are looking for.

Tina: Well, I obviously can't prove that I'll never meet the right guy. I just have had no success, so far.

Therapist: Right. Nobody can fully predict the future. Now, let's suppose that you acted badly or weakly and inadequately with the men in your life up till now. In what way does that – your poor behaviour – make you a weak and inadequate person?

Tina: That's how I've been up to now, always picking men who turn out to be the wrong type for me. Doesn't that prove that I'm weak and inadequate?

Therapist: Not to me, it doesn't! You may have *acted* weakly and inadequately with the men in your life, but how does it follow that you become a weak and inadequate *person*? You are a complex entity, a person who has performed many thousands or millions of acts in your lifetime, some good, some bad, some neutral. You also possess many traits, qualities and other aspects to your personality which change over time so long as you are alive. You can rate or evaluate your deeds, acts and performances according to some standard or goal. For example, you can rate your ability as a tennis player, but how can you give your 'self', your 'personhood' any kind of overall rating?

Tina: I don't know.

Therapist: You can't, is the answer. Let's see if I can explain this to you a little more clearly. I've a diagram that clients find very useful to help them remember this concept when they are feeling stressed out by some particular problem.[7] Would you like to see it?

Tina: Yes.

The therapist drew a big I on a whiteboard (Figure 7.2; see also Appendix 8).

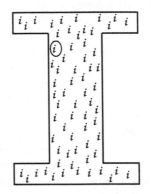

Figure 7.2 *The Big I/Little i diagram*

Therapist: Now, Tina, this big I represents you, your totality. And I'm going to fill it up in a minute with little 'i's which stand for various things about you, such as the way you smile, the kind of TV programme you like, and so on.

Tina: I get you.

Therapist: OK. Now let's fill in this big I with a few things about you.

Tina: I'm ready.

Therapist: Now, Tina, what would your family or friends say were some of your good points?

Tina: Oh, well, I've got a good sense of humour, and – let me see – I am kind-hearted, good to my children, I keep the house clean, I see that they're looked after properly ... will that do?

As Tina was speaking, the therapist began to draw a series of little 'i's inside the big I.

Therapist: Each of these little 'i's stands for some part of you, Tina; this one (pointing to a little 'i') stands for your good sense of humour, this other one stands for your kind-heartedness, and these other little 'i's represent all those other good points you mentioned you had.

Tina: I understand.

Therapist: Now, these are some of the positive things, the good things people might say about you. But what about your enemies? What sort of things might they say about you?

Tina: My enemies? Well, some would say I easily get angry, and I drive too fast sometimes ... and I'm too trusting ... .

Therapist: (writing more little 'i's inside the big I): ... Gets angry, drives too fast, too trusting. These are some of your not so good points.

Tina: Right.

Therapist: OK. Now what about neutral things? Give me a few things about you that are neither good nor bad.

Tina: Oh well, my dress sense isn't too bad, I suppose, and I can do alterations to the children's clothes that don't make them look too stitched up, and my house decorating ability is about average, I guess.

Therapist: (adding more little 'i's to represent Tina's neutral points): Right. Now, notice this, Tina. If we spent all day on this we'd end up with lots of little 'i's. In fact, if we considered *all* the things you've done since the day you were born – we couldn't really, of course, but just suppose we could – we'd have *millions* of little 'i's, all different aspects of yourself, good, bad and neutral, or neither good nor bad.

Tina: Yes, I see.

Therapist: Now, Tina, when you fail at something, like picking your ex-boyfriend and then finding you've made a bad choice (therapist now circles one little 'i' to denote this), you say 'Because I picked this partner and I made a poor choice yet again, that proves I'm a weak and inadequate person'. Are you actually being accurate?

Tina: Well, I did make a big mistake when I picked him, and that's the fourth time I've been dumped after picking the wrong guy! Once again I failed to pick somebody who was right for me.

Therapist: (pointing to the little 'i' he had circled inside the big I): Agreed. But how does that – this little 'i' – make *you* (pointing to the big I) a total failure, a weak and inadequate person? You failed to pick someone who would turn out to be the kind of partner you wanted; that is just one lIttle 'i'. And *you*, big I, consist of millions of little 'i's, right?

Tina: So my mistake, bad as it is, isn't the total me – is that what you're saying?

Therapist: Yes. Your mistake is only one *aspect* of *you*, just one little 'i' amongst millions of things you've done throughout your life so far. And consider this: we could go on and on filling up the big I with little 'i' after little 'i' because you are still alive, there are all your tomorrows and the new things you will do, and the changes in yourself. You, Tina, are not a static entity, but rather an ongoing, ever-changing process, too complex to ever be given any kind of overall or global rating such as good or bad, or a success or a failure.

Tina: So, I can't really rate my *self* – my big I, as you call it?

Therapist: Right. You can rate your performances, your skills, your acts. That is OK, because then you can identify your faults or shortcomings and try to correct them so that you do better. Philosophically speaking, you cannot legitimately rate your 'self' at all.

Tina: So, does that mean that I don't have to think of myself as a weak or inadequate *person* because I have *behaved* at times weakly or inadequately?

Therapist: That's right. *You*, the *person* known as Tina, are not the same thing as your *behaviour*. Your deeds, traits and performances are only *aspects* of you. Moreover, as a human you are fallible. We are all fallible. That's our nature. You've made mistakes in the past, and you'll almost certainly make more of them in the future. But you don't have to condemn *yourself* for your mistakes and errors. Accept yourself as having the right to be wrong, and try to learn from your mistakes so that you make fewer mistakes in future. You can be less wrong but never perfect. That's what being human means.

Tina: I'm entitled to make mistakes, errors of judgement where men are concerned, and things like that?

Therapist: Yes. We're not saying it's *right* to make mistakes, because it's certainly better or wiser not to. But as a fallible, screwed-up human individual, you'll inevitably make many errors. Because that's the way you are! You can train yourself to be more accepting of your own fallibility, and that goes for others' fallibility, including that of your ex-boyfriend.

Tina: Including my ex-boyfriend?

Therapist: Especially your ex-boyfriend! He sounds pretty screwed up to me, I don't know him, of course, but in view of what he has done to you, and the fact that he's into drugs, it looks like he's got a good many unresolved problems of his own. But he is still only a fallible, screwed-up human! So it makes good sense to accept others with their fallibilities as well as accepting yourself. Otherwise, how are you going to manage your life in a competent manner if you go through life, continually putting yourself down and hating others for your and their mistaken deeds or behaviour? That is the third major feature of Irrational Beliefs: they block you from achieving your goals. Their other two main characteristics, which we've just been discussing, are their illogicality, and the fact that they are not consistent with reality.

Tina: Hmm! That's a lot to remember. How do I change myself, then, and become a more sanely thinking person?

Therapist: By going over what we've been talking about many, many times. By Disputing your IBs until you really see that they make no sense, and learning to fully accept yourself and others as fallible. OK. The next time you fail at something, what will you do to remind yourself of these important concepts we've just been discussing?

Tina: No problem. I'll just remember this diagram.

Therapist: Good. Now, while we're about it, can you see how you made yourself feel angry and hurt over your boyfriend's poor behaviour?

Tina: Well, let me see. I probably created my own feelings of hurt and anger from my Irrational Beliefs.

Therapist: I pointed out that your hurt and anger sprang from your Irrational Belief, 'He *absolutely should* not have treated me in this unfair manner. And because he did treat me as he must not, he is a rotten person!' Is there any reason why he *absolutely should not* have treated you in that unfair manner?

Tina: Well, no. He did, didn't he? What happened, happened.

Therapist: Right. It would have been better if he had not treated you unfairly, but there is no reason why he absolutely should not have treated you unfairly. If he did, he did! That is the reality. Now what about the last part of the IB, 'And because he did treat me in that manner, he is a *rotten person*'?

Tina: Ah, let me see. He behaved rottenly by treating me the way he did, but that doesn't make him a rotten person?

Therapist: Right. Why doesn't it?

Tina: Because his rotten act is just one aspect of him, a little 'i', not his total self?

Therapist: Right, you're getting it! A rotten person would be a person who was rotten through and through, who had an *essence* of rottenness, and who could never be anything else but rotten for the rest of his life. Your ex may be screwed-up in various ways, and have a number of serious problems, but it is most unlikely that he is a totally rotten individual.

Tina: I guess that makes sense. I never want to see him again, but he has a right to live.

Therapist: All right. Now the final piece of information I'm going to give you is this: Whenever you get very upset, no matter what the circumstances, there is almost always in your head an absolute should, ought or must. The main forms they take are as follows: (a) 'I must do well, and be loved and approved by those who matter to me. If I'm not, it's awful, and I can't stand it and that proves I'm no good!'; (b) 'You must treat me fairly and nicely, and it's awful, and I can't stand it when you don't. You are no good for not treating me well, and deserve to be damned for doing what you must not do'; (c) 'The world must give me what I want quickly, without too much trouble or pain. If it doesn't, it's horrible, and life isn't worth living.'

Zero in on these Irrational Beliefs. They are there, not usually in the exact way I am stating them here, but in different words of your own which mean virtually the same thing. And you can find them, and Dispute them vigorously and persistently in your head and in other ways I will show you, until you give them up and replace them with more rational convictions.

Tina proved to be an apt pupil. She worked hard at identifying and disputing her Irrational Beliefs and eventually came up with an Effective New Philosophy or set of Rational Beliefs: 'I wish this betrayal of trust had not happened to me, but there is no reason why it must not. It is certainly unpleasant to be robbed of things that I valued, and both I and my children will be inconvenienced and faced with some degree of hardship as a result. But I can stand the unpleasantness and inconvenience of being deprived and I will do the best I can to help my children to get over this drawback. Although this is the fourth time I have been left by the men in my life, that only proves that I have not succeeded so far in finding the right kind of man for me. Even if I have made mistakes, that does not demean me in any way or prove that I am a weak or inadequate person. I accept myself and I can try to win a new relationship in due course with a reliable, trustworthy person and get him to accept me with my fallibility and shortcomings.

'As for my ex-boyfriend, he undoubtedly treated me badly, but there is no reason why he absolutely should not. He is not a rotten individual but a fallible human who probably has severe problems but is not a damnable person for having them.'

And her therapist then responded 'That's more like it. With these Rational Beliefs, you will feel sorry, displeased, annoyed and disappointed at the betrayal you experienced, but you won't feel depressed, enraged, self-pitying or in a mood to withdraw from all future contacts with men. You will also be motivated to see what constructive actions you can take to ameliorate your financial losses and maybe consider applying for better-paying jobs to help recoup the losses you suffered at the hands of your ex-boyfriend.'

Tina did, in fact, begin to improve her situation. She was loaned a serviceable secondhand TV from an old friend she had known from her schooldays; and she regularly studied the Situations Vacant columns of her local newspaper to see what jobs might offer her better prospects.

Since Tina was receptive to the REBT teaching she received as part of her treatment, no relaxation techniques were found to be necessary. She was, however, given information on nutrition and offered tips on how to get the best value for money in order to make the most of her limited resources.

Meanwhile, as part of her ongoing counselling sessions, her REBT therapist showed Tina how to use other cognitive and emotive-evocative techniques to reinforce the effects of the cognitive disputing she had been doing throughout her programme of stress reduction. She practised rational emotive imagery, by letting herself feel outraged and horrified, as she imagined being betrayed by a lover again. She then changed these unhealthy negative feelings to healthy negative emotions of sorrow, annoyance and disappointment. Then she practised new rational coping statements to keep replacing her unhealthy feelings of horror with her healthier self-helping feelings.

Tina tape-recorded sessions with her therapist in which he played the devil's advocate and attempted to talk Tina out of her Rational Beliefs, while she defended them. Then he critiqued her efforts.

Tina recorded forceful self-dialogues with herself in which she played both her Irrational Voice and her Rational Voice. In her Irrational Voice, Tina rehearsed all the arguments she could think of in support of her Irrational Beliefs and against her Rational Beliefs. Then, speaking in her Rational Voice, she answered the arguments of her Irrational Voice one by one, and in a very forceful manner, until her Irrational Voice conceded defeat. The therapist then critiqued her efforts.[8]

Once her therapist was satisfied that Tina had begun to internalize her Rational Beliefs and held them strongly instead of lightly or weakly, he gave her some assertion training. He suspected that in her previous relationships, Tina had been too eager to please the men she met and dated, and as a consequence had insufficiently attended to her own preferences and priorities. She had read in a magazine somewhere that men didn't like 'pushy' women and that the best strategy for winning a boyfriend was to be nice, uncritical and accommodating, otherwise she would be overlooked for women whom men found less trouble to date. Her therapist was sceptical of these notions and showed her how to make a list of all the advantages of taking risks and getting, probably, many rejections while doing so, and all the disadvantages of 'comfortably' refusing to take such risks and waiting like a sitting duck for personable men to come to her.[9]

She role-played with the therapist methods of encountering men and talking to them in a sustained manner without feeling obliged to fall in with their wishes unless and until she felt ready and really wanted to.

Cognitively, she learned to use REBT self-questioning to rip up the idea that she needed a man to 'validate her as a woman'. She eventually convinced herself that she did not have to find love; that it wasn't a catastrophe if she didn't find it; that she could stand rejection; and that the more she risked encountering men, the better her chances would be of finding a suitable man.

Tina's homework assignments included bibliotherapy materials to read on how to go about encountering and dating men, such as Ellis's *The Intelligent Woman's Guide to Dating and Mating* and *A New Guide to Rational Living*.[10]

She was also given shame-attacking exercises such as encountering men and deliberately saying the wrong thing while accepting herself and showing herself how to refuse to down herself while she did so.

Behaviourally, Tina took the assignment of encountering each month a few possible love partners. By getting mainly rejected by them, she became desensitized to rejection, did not feel ashamed or self-pitying, nor did she feel obliged to go along with the demands of the men she met.

Tina terminated counselling after 16 sessions with her REBT therapist. By then she had overcome her original problem, for which she received crisis intervention. Since then she has demonstrated a satisfactory level of competence in effectively managing her life and relating well to a man with whom she now shares her household.

Time-limited brief therapy

Time-limited brief therapy is a special case of brief therapy. Occasionally a client may request stress counselling to help her cope with an unexpected crisis or to ameliorate severe anxiety about some forthcoming event in the immediate future. Severe time limitations may thus constrain your client to just a single session of stress counselling. If your client mentions she has more than one problem, it may be advisable to prioritize her problems and to deal with the most urgent one first in view of the limited time available in a single session – usually one to two hours. If the client agrees, her less urgent problems may be scheduled for discussion at a later date. In exceptionally severe cases, McMullin recommends a four-hour marathon session if feasible, in which you spend up to four hours teaching your client cognitive methods in a very active-directive manner without breaks until your client comprehends how to use your distress combating techniques.[11]

Subject to the usual contraindications, some clients may benefit from relaxation prior to receiving REBT. Other severely anxious clients may benefit more from relaxation with hypnosis followed by a powerful REBT message designed to counteract their anxiety. The entire period of relaxation and hypnosis with REBT may be recorded on an audiocassette and given to clients to take home and listen to at least once before they are due to face the anxiety-provoking situation. Useful examples of scripts for carrying out multimodal relaxation and hypnosis stage by stage can be found in Stephen Palmer's book *Multimodal Techniques: Relaxation and Hypnosis*. The hypnosis script may be targeted at specific symptoms the client may be suffering from, including allergies, anxiety, asthma, habits the client wishes to change (e.g. overeating, smoking), insomnia and various other ailments. (For a description of Palmer's MRM script refer back to Chapter 6, page 85.) Caution should be exercised before using these techniques to ensure that no organic condition is present if treatment is directed towards symptom removal. You need also to be aware of the contraindications of relaxation techniques which are outlined in Palmer's book.[12]

Single-session stress counselling with Jane

We recommend that you have a preliminary telephone conversation with the potential client before confirming an appointment to ensure the client's time is not wasted. This has several advantages:

1. You may be able to ascertain exactly what your client is most distressed about.
2. You may have the opportunity to explain briefly to your client the rationale of REBT counselling and how this may help to reduce her level of distress and help her to manage her problem more effectively.
3. If there are no contraindications, you may then explain to your client that you envisage up to two hours of single-session counselling being necessary to help her with her problem. If she agrees to try your approach and to set aside the necessary time, you may arrange an appointment.

Palmer and Dryden list seven conditions that may, but won't necessarily, contraindicate brief therapy. There are no rigid rules in the matter, and here, as elsewhere, a counsellor's clinical experience and acumen are the best guide to deciding whether or not a given client can benefit from single-session stress counselling.[13]

In Jane's case there were no contraindications and as she seemed willing to try REBT without prior relaxation, her therapist considered her a suitable candidate for a single session of stress counselling.

ASSESSMENT AND TREATMENT

Jane described her reasons for seeking stress counselling as:

> I won promotion to my present position only a few weeks ago and very soon I have to give a 10-minute presentation to my Board of directors. I've never done anything like this before and I'm absolutely petrified at the prospect! It's important for my future prospects in the company that I make a good impression on the Board, especially since it will be my first attempt. But I feel so anxious about giving a good presentation that I can hardly think of anything else. I find it difficult to concentrate on my work, and I'm not sleeping well for constantly thinking about it.

One of your aims at the assessment stage is to arrive as quickly as possible at the 'critical A', that is, that part of the Activating Event that triggers off Jane's Irrational Beliefs that lead to her feeling anxious. The form on page 119 is designed to achieve this and has already been filled in to illustrate how it was used in this particular case. Since it can also be used by clients as part of a homework assignment, a blank version appears in Appendix 5.

The form on page 119 has been designed to facilitate inference chaining, as the example indicates. As indicated, her critical A was 'Giving a poor presentation to the Board'.

Jane's first task was to learn the ABCDE model. Once your client understands the connection between A, B and C, you may help her identify her core Irrational

Workplace Problem (A)	Self-Defeating Beliefs (B)	Emotional/ Behavioural Consequences (C)	Disputing Self-Defeating Beliefs (D)	New Effective Approach to Problem (E)
Giving a presentation to the Board of Directors	'I must give a good presentation otherwise the outcome will be awful'	Anxious; difficulty in concentrating on work; not sleeping well	Logical: Just because I want to give a good presentation, how does it logically follow that I must give a good presentation?	Although it's strongly preferable to give a good presentation, I don't have to.
Giving a poor presentation to the Board (critical A)			Empirical: Where is the evidence that my demand must be granted?	There is no evidence that I will get what I demand even if it is preferable and desirable.
I might lose my job			Am I being realistic? If I don't give a good presentation will the outcome really be awful?	If I don't give a good presentation, the outcome may be bad, but hardly awful and the end of the world!
I would have to sell my apartment			Pragmatic: Where is it getting me holding on to this belief?	If I continue holding on to this belief, I will remain very anxious and even more likely to give a poor presentation.
				If I change my attitude I will feel concerned and not anxious. Also I will be able to concentrate and prepare for the lecture. My sleeping will probably improve too and I'll feel refreshed. I'll ensure that I practise Rational Emotive Imagery to overcome my anxiety.

Beliefs. In Jane's case her core IB was: 'I must give a good presentation otherwise the outcome will be awful.' This was entered in column B. Once Jane understood that B, her Irrational Belief, and not A, giving a poor presentation to the Board, mainly created her anxious feelings and inability to concentrate on her work at C, she then proceeded to column D where she was shown how to Dispute her IBs, using the three main strategies: the logical, the empirical and the pragmatic. Finally, Jane replaces her IBs with Rational Beliefs (RBs). The RBs Jane came up with are shown in column E.

The therapist explained to Jane that her more Rational Beliefs about giving a presentation to the Board will lead her to feel healthy concern, rather than crippling anxiety, about doing well, and will motivate her to concentrate on presenting her case to the best of her ability.

Once Jane had replaced her IBs with the Rational Beliefs (RBs) shown in column E, the therapist suggested methods she could use to help reinforce her new more rational attitude. Jane was shown how to use rational-emotive imagery in which she let herself feel anxious as she imagined herself doing poorly in her presentation, and then changing these unhealthy negative feelings to a healthy negative emotion of concern. Then she practised forceful coping statements to keep replacing her unhealthy feelings of anxiety with healthier self-helping feelings of concern and a strong desire to do her best. As time permitted a small amount of bibliotherapy, Jane was given a copy of Michael Neenan's succinct paper, 'An introduction to rational emotive behaviour therapy' (see Appendix 6), which showed her how to tackle a problem of performance anxiety over public speaking quite similar to her own. Finally, the therapist suggested that if time allowed, she could record her proposed ten-minute presentation to the Board on an audio-cassette and arrange for him or some other counsellor to listen to it and critique her efforts.

OUTCOME

Jane did manage to give a satisfactory presentation. She reported that she felt quite nervous as she began her presentation, but by focusing on what she wanted to say and by concentrating on how she had decided to present her case, her nervousness subsided and she felt good about the way her presentation was received and the comments she received afterwards from one of the Board members.

In this example the client was able to control her anxiety to the level which enabled her to give a satisfactory presentation to the Board. That was her immediate problem and the entire session was devoted to helping her to resolve it. Since clients will often have other less pressing problems they may wish to resolve, they may feel encouraged by their first success in using REBT to ask you for more extended counselling to deal with their other problems. You may then welcome the opportunity this affords you to deepen and strengthen their emerging more rational attitude, and help them realize their potential for achieving a more profound philosophic change.

Bearing in mind the indications and contraindications of brief therapy, time-limited sessions play a useful part in the repertoire of counselling techniques by giving clients with urgent problems the opportunity to acquire the means to cope with their problems which otherwise would remain unresolved.

NOTES

1. Palmer and Ellis, 1995a.
2. Dryden, 1995b.
3. McMullin, 1986.
4. Dryden, 1995b, p. 8.
5. Ellis, 1996.
6. Palmer and Dryden, 1995.
7. Lazarus, 1977.
8. Dryden, 1995b; Ellis, 1992a, 1994b, 1996.
9. Ellis, 1985b, p. 43.
10. Ellis, 1979c; Ellis and Harper, 1975, 1997.
11. McMullin, 1986.
12. Palmer, 1993d.
13. Palmer and Dryden, 1995, p. 200.

CHAPTER 8

How to Deal with Difficult Clients

The bold title of this chapter is not meant to claim surefire methods of overcoming the sort of problems that difficult clients usually present, but to offer a few techniques and strategies that may prove effective with this client group. The term 'difficult clients' refers to those individuals whose level of disturbance, of innate or acquired deficiencies, of resistance or even sheer bloody-mindedness hinders them from engaging in and benefiting from therapy. REBT practitioners frequently refer to such clients as DCs (difficult customers) or TCs (tough customers). Such descriptions are not used to disparage clients but to alert you to the hard work and determination required to effect some amelioration in these clients' emotional and behavioural problems. DCs often present a formidable challenge to your ability to help them.

Different REBT therapists emphasize different groups of DCs. Ellis and Dryden describe them as '... individuals who are in the psychotic, borderline, organic, or mental deficient category' while Young includes '... individuals from lower socio-economic classes, uncooperative adolescents, Fundamentalist Christians, and those with limited intelligence'.[1] One of the individuals left out of the foregoing groups and who often impedes or undermines the progress of therapy is the therapist. Ellis observes that 'although the literature on difficult and resistant clients is extensive ... much less attention has been given to the difficult and resistant therapist'. On the theme of resistance in therapy, Ellis asserts that 'overcoming clients' resistance to therapeutic change is in some ways the most important problem in psychotherapy'.[2]

REBT's multimodal (cognitive, emotive, behavioural, imaginal) approach to therapy uses active persuasion as well as force and energy to motivate, encourage and push difficult clients to look at their resistance and to commit themselves to therapy in order for them to achieve some measure of constructive change.

CLIENT RESISTANCE

Fear of discomfort

Clients frequently resist changing because of their fear of discomfort. They view the change process as *too* hard and *too* uncomfortable to endure, and thereby create low frustration tolerance (LFT). If some of your clients have LFT about changing, you can repeatedly and strongly show them that avoiding hard work *now* will actually increase their problems later and make their life conditions even more difficult to cope with. Show them, again, 'no matter how hard it is for you to change, it's distinctly harder if you don't'. Their philosophy of short-range hedonism, i.e. often seeking immediate gratification and avoiding pain and discomfort, keeps them mired in the present and myopic about the future.[3] Urge your clients to attack vigorously their LFT-producing Beliefs about change, e.g. 'I *can't stand* all the hassle I'll have to go through!' Help them to try a system of rewards and penalties when, respectively, they carry out therapeutic tasks and when they do not. Through these activities it is more likely clients will develop a philosophy of effort ('There's no gain without pain') that leads to long-range hedonism, i.e. enjoying the pleasures of the moment as well as planning constructively for the future (now that they see they have one).

Fear of disclosure and shame

Your clients may feel that if they reveal 'shameful' thoughts or actions – e.g. masturbating while looking at a pornographic magazine – you, their therapist, may condemn them. But reluctance to talk about such problems, of course, perpetuates the emotional distress they are seeking help to overcome. You can help them minimize this kind of resistance by offering them unconditional acceptance and by revealing and challenging their Irrational Beliefs (IBs), e.g. 'I must not behave in such a disgusting way. If my therapist discovers this about me he will think how worthless I am.' You can teach them to give themselves unconditional self-acceptance (USA) so that they are hardly ever ashamed to tell you any of their 'disgusting' behaviours.

Fear of change or success

Your clients' process of change can lead to unpredictable and frightening consequences, so they conclude that it is safer to stay with the discomfort they are familiar with rather than venture into the unknown. Clients are not usually afraid of success itself but of the subsequent failure that may easily occur after initial success. If this is so, identify, challenge and change the fear-inducing beliefs of your clients, e.g. 'I won't be able to bear all the upheavals in my life if I start changing things'. 'If I start to improve my life it may well fall apart later anyway. That would be awful!'

By removing the 'horror' (emotional disturbance) from the often painful process of change, you can teach your clients to habituate themselves to new ways and to realistically evaluate how 'overwhelmed' they actually are. Stepping out from the false security of their 'comfort of discomfort', they can accept risk-taking and uncertainty as the inevitable consequences of seeking a more rewarding life. They can learn to refrain from labelling themselves as *failures* because of their particular *failings*. As Paul Hauck notes, instead of self-downing, they can develop self-efficacy or achievement-confidence because by taking chances '... you learn something from your attempt – even if it's only what not to do next time – and you use that knowledge in your next trial. That's not failure. It's gradual success and that's impossible without risk-taking.'[4]

THERAPIST RESISTANCE

Therapists disturb themselves in similar ways to their clients by holding absolutist beliefs that can impede or undermine their clients' progress. Ellis has advanced several Irrational Beliefs that he believes lead to therapeutic inefficiency. These include: 'I have to be successful with all my clients practically all the time.' 'I must be an outstanding therapist, clearly better than other therapists I know or hear about.' 'I have to be greatly respected and loved by all my clients.'[5]

How can therapists become aware they are holding such dysfunctional Beliefs? Dryden advises them ' ... to monitor your feelings and behaviours, and use these as a guide to the detection of your therapy-related irrational beliefs'.[6] For example, if you become anxious about confronting a client's repeated excuses for not doing her homework tasks because you fear losing her approval, your IB may be 'I must have her approval in order to see myself as a competent therapist'. By carrying out the ABCDE method of self-analysis and change, you can remove your own disturbance-producing beliefs and give yourself the homework task of encouraging your client, in the above example, to carry out her homework.

Ellis actually urges therapists to wrestle with their problems on their own rather than seek immediate help because '... you may be able to appreciate better the struggles of your own clients when they strive for self-change; and you may thereby come to accept them with their struggles and setbacks'.[7] If you are still unable to overcome your self-created blocks to doing effective therapy, you can tackle them by getting some supervision or through personal therapy.

Hauck identified another form of therapist disturbance which he called 'the neurotic agreement in psychotherapy'.[8] In this case, the therapist's failure to challenge the client's irrational ideas may stem from her own adherence to the same beliefs, e.g. 'I *absolutely must* have a partner in my life in order to be worthwhile'. Such a 'neurotic agreement' will leave unexamined important problems of your client unless you first discover and dispute your own Irrational Beliefs.

SUBSTANCE ABUSE

REBT hypothesizes that the '... primary cognitive dynamic that creates and maintains addiction is what we call the abstinence LFT pattern'.[9] Addicted individuals often devoutly believe that they must have an enjoyable substance, such as alcohol or cocaine, because 'I *must* not be deprived' or, when they feel distressed, they insist 'I can't stand this stress and must cover it up with alcohol, food, or some other distracting substance!' So most addicts have severe 'discomfort anxiety' or LFT. Working with addicts is doubly difficult because their LFT beliefs not only usually encourage a quick return to substance abuse to ease their discomfort anxiety, but also militate against the hard work required to change addictive behaviour, especially learning how to tackle their disturbed feelings such as depression and anger, that frequently help to drive them to addictions.[10]

You can help addicted clients to construct vigorous coping self-statements to combat their LFT beliefs – such as 'I hate my bloody anxious feelings, but I can stand them!' You can also teach your clients to develop forceful self-dialogues in the course of which they vigorously convince themselves of the real disadvantages of abusing alcohol, drugs or other substances. As a therapist, see that your clients' arguments against further addictions are more convincing than those for it.

Those cognitive techniques can be coupled with stimulus control, i.e. avoiding or reducing exposure to situations that may trigger substance abuse such as visiting certain friends or areas of town. Greenwood suggests that stimulus control is '... a quick way for people to gain some control over substance abuse behavior ...'.[11] Once clients have achieved some stability in their lives, they can focus on and tackle the original reasons for their abusing drink and/or drugs, frequently their perceived inability to cope with failure or rejection and their consequent self-denigration.

Relapse prevention is also part of REBT therapy. If your clients do return to drink or drugs, you had better focus primarily on their dysfunctional ideas and behaviours leading up to the relapse. They also often have secondary symptoms, e.g. guilt and shame, about 'falling off the wagon'. That makes them feel like *rotten persons* who 'cannot' act well and return to sobriety. So help them accept themselves *with* their relapsing, and then to think and act differently to return to recovery.

In my work with drug users, I (M.N.) find that many clients resist the REBT concept of emotional responsibility, i.e. that they are primarily responsible for their emotional and behavioural reactions to life events. In REBT parlance, instead of using B–C thinking, they blame external events or others for their problems (A–C thinking). In popular parlance, they unrealistically view reality in terms of 'It does my head in'. They mean that an infinite variety of problems and pressures – and not their *reactions* to these stressors – do them in. You can teach them emotional responsibility by using the ABC model, 'How do you *let* "it" do your head in?' By contradicting their view of themselves as, for example, 'helpless' or an 'addictive personality', you can help them make a perceptual shift that serves as a catalyst for change in their lives.

In addition to therapy, clients may require a supervised detoxification programme from such substances as alcohol, heroin or tranquillizers. Long-term or chaotic substance abusers often need prolonged in-patient detox/rehabilitation treatment to prepare themselves for drug-free living.

POST-TRAUMATIC STRESS DISORDER

Post-traumatic stress disorder (PTSD) refers to '... the development of characteristic symptoms following exposure to an extreme traumatic stressor ...'.[12] Traumatic events include combat experiences, earthquakes, rapes, violent assaults, car crashes, etc. PTSD reactions involve, among other symptoms, intrusive recollections of the event, sleep disturbances, avoidance behaviour, exaggerated startle response, outbursts of anger, hypervigilance, emotional numbing and flashbacks to the original trauma. Warren and Zgourides suggest that education about PTSD is an important part of therapy and therefore '... advocate teaching clients a conceptual model that clearly explains the development of PTSD symptoms. Such a conceptual framework, in and of itself, should aid in bringing some order to the client's sense of chaos.'[13]

REBT writers, such as Ellis and Moore, agree with Janoff-Bulman that individuals' rigid, overly confident and unexamined pre-trauma beliefs and assumptions about themselves, others and the world are more likely to be shattered by the trauma than beliefs and assumptions which are more realistic and adaptable to adversity in life.[14] Pre-trauma unrealistic beliefs and assumptions include *personal invulnerability*, e.g. 'Nothing terrible will ever happen to me'; *self-worth*, e.g. 'I must see myself as strong and competent in everything I do'; *fairness and justness in life*, e.g. 'If I'm kind and helpful to others then nothing bad or nasty should happen to me'. When traumatic events help to shatter these unreasonable assumptions, individuals often feel helpless, vulnerable, out of control, victimized, worthless. Secondary emotional disturbances frequently arise from the primary trauma as when a woman severely berates herself for not coping better with her PTSD symptoms.

You can use cognitive restructuring or rebuilding victims' shattered assumptions by encouraging them to examine their basic beliefs in order to introduce flexibility and realism into them. For example: 'I now realize that I'm not invulnerable to crime and had better be more safety conscious without becoming a prisoner in my own home.' 'I'm not weak and useless because I was temporarily careless about my personal safety. I can accept myself for my carelessness but will endeavour to be more careful in future.' 'Kindness to others is no guarantee of protection from nasty things in life. I might be mugged again but this possibility is not going to make me cynical or less charitable towards others.' Secondary disturbances can be tackled, as in the above example, by teaching the client to unconditionally accept rather than berate herself and thereby focus more on her energy on productive problem-solving rather than self-downing.

You can also facilitate rational philosophies and emotional change by using prolonged imaginal exposure to the original trauma (e.g. being mugged) and *in vivo* desensitization to presently avoided fearful situations (e.g. being out alone at night). By exposing clients to painful images and reminders of the trauma as well as discussing associated cognitive material (e.g. 'It's my fault I was mugged'), you can help them therapeutically accept such grim events and integrate these events into their lives. Other techniques you can use to help clients develop a greater sense of self-control and confidence include controlled breathing, muscle relaxation, thought stopping, assertion training, covert modelling (imagining anxiety-provoking situations and using coping strategies to tackle them successfully). Muran and DiGiuseppe suggest that working with '... PTSD client[s] requires a fine balance between empathy and support on one hand and encouragement and faith in the survivor's ability on the other hand'.[15]

OBSESSIVE COMPULSIVE DISORDER

Obsessive compulsive disorder (OCD) can be seen as one of the most disabling of the anxiety disorders.[16] Individuals with this condition have persistent and intrusive thoughts, images or impulses, e.g. 'Did I lock the front door?' (obsession) and repetitive behaviours, e.g. repeatedly checking the front door (compulsion). Anxiety-inducing obsessions are countered or neutralized (temporarily) by the compulsions.

Ellis hypothesizes that OCs (obsessive compulsives) tend to have biological deficits including: cognitive, e.g. overfocusing handicaps; emotive, e.g. affective overactivity; behavioural, e.g. compulsiveness. OCs exacerbate their deficits by developing low frustration tolerance (LFT) about them and condemning themselves for having these problems in the first place; in addition, they frequently develop secondary emotional problems (e.g. depression) in relation to their OCD. OCs are also prone to self-denigration and LFT over non-OCD related frustrations and failures in their lives. Such a catalogue of problems and the usually considerable persistence to effect therapeutic change leads Ellis to call many of them VDCs (very difficult customers).[17]

Principal treatment methods of OCD include exposure, response prevention and vigorous disputing of OCD-related Irrational Beliefs. You can expose the client to her anxiety regarding, as in the above example, the 'awful' consequences of an unlocked front door and encourage her to refrain from engaging in the usual anxiety-reducing ritual of checking – this is the response prevention aspect. At the same time, she targets her dogmatic demands for disputing, e.g. 'I must check my front door 30 times before I go to work to make sure it's safe and secure. I *can't stand* the agony of not checking and the hardship and misery my life will undergo if I fail to check and my house is burgled.' She is also urged not to seek reassurance (another form of neutralizing) from others, e.g. family, friends, work colleagues, therapist, that nothing bad will happen because she only checked once. These various methods are designed to achieve habituation to her anxiety and discomfort and enable her to evaluate realistically whether the feared consequences of not repeatedly checking will actually occur.

You can help neutralize some clients' obsessional thoughts which are accompanied by covert cognitive rituals rather than overt behavioural ones. For example, 'I must kill my wife' is countered by 'I love my wife'. On these occasions, habituation to obsessions can be achieved by such methods as the client listening continuously to his recorded intrusive thoughts on a loop tape. Response prevention to the neutralizing thought can be tackled with thought-stopping or distraction techniques.[18]

Dryden states that guilt plays an important role in OCD as clients assume excessive responsibility for the harm that might befall themselves or others through things done or omitted, or feel wicked for having thoughts such as a mother imagining harming her child. Clients are taught to distinguish between labelling their thoughts and behaviours as 'bad' or 'wicked' (if they choose to see them in this way) and avoiding condemning themselves for having these thoughts or actions.[19] Clients can be challenged on their overestimate of how much responsibility they actually have in causing harm to others, e.g. '... the crime rate would be much higher than it is if obsessive thoughts lead to harming others'.[20] You can show clients that they do not have total control over their thinking in their attempts to stop their wicked thoughts, e.g. you tell the client that she must not think of a bright red car but she is unable to follow your instructions. This demonstrates that the more she tries to control her forbidden thoughts their frequency only increases.

Ellis stresses that teaching clients unconditional self-acceptance in the face of their manifold problems and the use of the techniques already described (though these are hardly all of them) can '... help clients reduce and minimize, but rarely entirely eliminate, their OCD behaviours'.[21]

PERSONALITY DISORDERS

Young and Lindemann advance two important characteristics of clients with personality disorders: '... first is the presence of enduring, inflexible traits ...' and second the avoidance '... of painful memories, associations, and feelings'. Disturbed interpersonal relationships may be offered as a third characteristic.[22] Because of the long-standing nature of their characterological problems, Beck, Freeman and Associates suggest '... they are often the most difficult patients in a clinician's case-load. They generally require more work within the session, longer time for therapy, greater strain on the therapist's skills (and patience), and more therapist energy than do most other patients.'[23] Examples of personality disorder and the corresponding basic beliefs include: narcissistic – 'I am a very special person'; dependent – 'I am helpless'; paranoid – 'I cannot trust other people'; avoidant – 'I may get terribly hurt'.

The REBT literature on personality disorders has focused in particular on the borderline personality.[24] Borderline personality disorder is defined in DSM-IV as 'a pervasive pattern of instability of interpersonal relationships, self-image, and affects, and marked impulsivity beginning by early childhood and present in a variety of contexts ...'[25] Ellis hypothesizes that borderline personalities have innate cognitive (e.g. rigid ways of thinking, attention deficits), emotive (e.g. overexcitable, highly-strung) and behavioural (e.g. hyperactive, impulsive) deficits which they largely inherit. Added to these existing problems, such individuals may severely condemn themselves and exhibit low frustration tolerance (LFT) on the basis of these deficits which, in turn, leads to further emotional disturbance.[26]

Ellis suggests that therapists establish a warm, supportive but usually firm therapeutic manner which offers clients unconditional acceptance as fallible human beings, but not always of their behaviours, e.g. frequent temper tantrums, demands for non-scheduled 'crisis' sessions, frequent changes of therapeutic goals, not carrying out their negotiated homework tasks.[27] It is important to provide feedback to clients on the self-defeating nature of their thoughts, feelings and behaviours without displaying your own anger or sense of hopelessness about these blocks and frustrations. You can also strive to teach clients to accept themselves with their multifarious problems including '... that he or she has certain inflexible personality traits'.[28] When clients become easily frustrated or despondent over lack of progress, Ellis exhorts therapists to 'Encourage, encourage, encourage! Show your clients that you know that they can change – and keep firmly, patiently pushing them to do so.'[29]

You can identify rigid ways of thinking, e.g. 'I'm utterly worthless', 'I'll never be able to change', 'Everyone lets me down' to show them that such all or nothing thinking significantly contributes to their problems. Through showing clients how to examine such beliefs, you can help them to learn to develop more self-helping ways of viewing themselves and others. For example, 'If I can learn to separate my actions from myself, I won't put myself down so often'; 'I can change, even just a little, with hard work as I showed by doing my homework task'; 'People do let me down but not all of the time'. Along with cognitive modification, Ellis emphasizes that skill training (e.g. improving impulse control) '... is almost mandatory with many of them [borderlines]'.[30]

By such methods, among others, clients can learn to develop greater emotional and behavioural control in their lives which, in turn, may bring a more stable and positive self-image though '... we can rarely help them achieve what may be called a "real" cure ... [of] their borderline condition'.[31]

EATING DISORDERS

The two major eating disorders are anorexia nervosa and bulimia nervosa. Bresler suggests that approximately 90 per cent of clients with these disorders are women. Onset of these disorders usually occurs in late adolescence or early adulthood; anorexia can be triggered by a stressful life event such as leaving home, while bulimia often begins during or after a period of dieting.[32]

Anorexia nervosa

The key features of this disorder '... are that the individual refuses to maintain a minimally normal body weight, is intensely afraid of gaining weight, and exhibits a significant disturbance in the perception of the shape or size of his or her body'.[33] Drastic dieting or semi-starvation regimes coupled with other weight control methods (e.g. self-induced vomiting) usually lead to medical complications such as electrolyte imbalances, impaired renal function, cardiovascular problems and osteoporosis. Associated mental problems include depressive and obsessive-compulsive symptoms.

As with bulimics, anorexic clients' core concern is judging '... their self-worth or value almost exclusively in terms of their shape and weight'.[34] Ellis states that his anorexic clients '... almost always *brought* perfectionist ideas to family situations and dogmatically held that they *had* to be completely thin to be worthwhile'. Other rigidly held ideas include equating self-discipline or control with weight loss, and weight gain ('fatness') with failure and repulsiveness. Ellis suggests that anorexic clients largely construct their eating disorders by bringing such irrational ideas to family and general life situations.[35]

Depending on the severity of the presenting symptoms, treatment is conducted on an in- or out-patient basis or a combination of the two over a period of time. Anorexic clients may be unaware of the serious consequences of their drastic dieting and therefore considerable therapist persistence will often be needed to overcome this problem. This can be coupled with education about anorexia. You can initiate a weight restoration programme to return clients to physical health as well as '... to enable them to engage effectively in psychological treatments designed to address these more central problems [anorexia-inducing irrational ideas]'.[36] Given the serious problems in dealing with eating disorders, Bresler emphasizes that non-medical therapists must work in conjunction with doctors, nurses, nutritionists and others familiar with these conditions.[37]

Your clients' core beliefs can be carefully examined and challenged. They can be taught the perils of self-esteem (e.g. 'I'm acceptable because I'm thin') and the benefits of unconditional self-acceptance: refusing to rate themselves on the basis of any particular trait or action but sensibly rating their behaviours, e.g. rating their strong desire for healthy slimness as good.

You can point out that discontent rather than disturbance about our bodies can be a healthy human reaction. Clients can look at the short- and long-term advantages and disadvantages of their preoccupation with thinness, e.g. they are missing out on alternative sources of satisfaction in their lives. By insisting on unrealistic total control of their body weight they are failing to develop a realistic sense of general control over their lives.

Clients' anxieties regarding weight gain, e.g. 'I'll become so fat and lose control of everything. It will be awful', can be 'de-awfulized' by clients imagining themselves reducing their excessive weight and thereby re-establishing self-control. They can also examine cultural propaganda that equates thinness with attractiveness and success and decide if they want to continue to believe it. Graded behavioural tasks can be undertaken to challenge irrational ideas, e.g. stopping exercise will result in massive weight gain.[38] Realistic perceptions of body image can be obtained by accepting '... the opinions of trusted others and on the basis of the information provided by weekly weighing'.[39]

By helping your client to challenge her self-defeating beliefs and to embrace self-acceptance, you can encourage her to learn '... to tolerate imperfection and discomfort that will give her the courage to risk expanding her repertoire of behaviours, and embarking on a more satisfying course of development'.[40]

Bulimia nervosa

The essential features of this disorder '... are binge eating and inappropriate compensatory methods [e.g. self-induced vomiting; misuse of laxatives or diuretics] to prevent weight gain'.[41] Binge eating is usually carried out in secret and is triggered by, among other things, unpleasant feelings, interpersonal difficulties and hunger through strict dieting. Dieting, bingeing and purging cycles are often accompanied by feelings of shame, guilt and the fear of being 'found out'. Like anorexics, bulimics may be preoccupied with or obsessed about their weight and shape and link these issues to their level of self-esteem. Medical complications of this disorder include electrolyte imbalances, dental damage, menstrual irregularities, metabolic problems.

You can use similar techniques with bulimics as you use with anorexics, e.g. education about the disorder including the general ineffectiveness of vomiting and purging as '... they [clients] cannot bring up all their food, or that laxatives have no effect whatsoever on absorption of calories'.[42] Also, establishing healthy eating patterns and giving up dieting; challenging their self-defeating ideas about body shape and weight; striving for self-acceptance rather than self-esteem; examining cultural notions of the 'beautiful body'.

Woods and Grieger present a complex ABC chain of bulimic behaviour as an analysis of how such behaviour is initiated and maintained, e.g. a woman becomes depressed over her 'obscene fatness', temporarily assuages her unhappiness with binge eating, then becomes desperate to get rid of the unwanted calories through laxative use, feels guilt and shame over her bingeing and purging, ameliorates these feelings and regains a sense of control through a return to strict dieting ... until the cycle starts again.[43]

Dryden recommends that clients intervene early in these complex chains to prevent the build-up of overwhelming disturbed feelings and counterproductive behaviours which will inhibit constructive problem-solving. Disturbance-producing beliefs in the chain are identified and challenged, e.g. 'Why must you be thin in order to be approved of?'; 'Is it realistic to state that thinness equals happiness?'; 'Where is it going to get you if you are always in fear of putting on weight?'; 'Let's devise a few experiments to determine if you can actually stand looking at your own body'.[44]

You can also institute stimulus control measures and other interventions, e.g. reducing emotional disturbance with REBT rather than food; suppressing hunger with low calorie snacks; removing or avoiding food temptations; eating slowly; throwing away leftovers; rewards and penalties for, respectively, healthy and unhealthy eating patterns. The long-term goal of treatment is to achieve weight stability and increased happiness through significant attitudinal and lifestyle changes.

PANIC DISORDER

The essential feature of this disorder '... is the presence of recurrent, unexpected panic attacks followed by at least 1 month of persistent concern about having another panic attack, worry about the possible implications or consequences of the panic attacks, or a significant behavioural change related to the attacks'.[45] Panic attack symptoms include pounding heart, trembling, hot flushes, shortness of breath, nausea, lightheadedness, fear of dying. Panic disorder may be accompanied by agoraphobia.

You can use education as a first step in treatment with clients learning a cognitive model of panic. This model suggests that triggering stimuli, e.g. dizziness (internal) or a social occasion (external) produce '... mild sensations which, once noticed, are interpreted in a catastrophic fashion. This interpretation produces a marked increase in anxiety, which leads to a further increase in bodily sensations and hence creates a vicious circle which culminates in an attack.'[46] The aim of therapy is to break this vicious circle.

Using the REBT perspective of a cognitive model, you can seek to elicit the inferences and their implicit demands in the build-up of panic.[47] For example, a client who is feeling apprehensive might construct the following inference-evaluative belief chain:

Inference – I'm going to have a heart attack.

↓

Irrational Belief – I must not have a heart attack!

↓

Inference – My heart is pounding so hard it's going to explode.

↓

Irrational Belief – I must be able to slow it down now!

↓

Inference – It's out of control. I'm going to die.

↓

Irrational Belief – I must not die like this! Somebody help me!

↓

Emotional Consequence – Panic

While REBT therapists usually look for the client's most clinically relevant inference (critical A) which 'springs' the disturbance-producing belief, when working with panic disorder your strategy can be to '... first help clients to understand how their irrational beliefs that occur earlier in the chain actually produce their increasingly distorted inferences later in the chain and then to help them to dispute these evaluative beliefs'.[48] If this intervention can be carried out while your client is experiencing incipient panic, it can prove to be a powerful method for defusing his or her impending sense of catastrophe.

You can dispute clients' ultimate fears, such as dying, losing control or going mad, along the lines of 'Why absolutely must it not occur?' You then help to remove the 'horror' (emotional disturbance) from their awfulizing about these things. If clients are not receptive to this philosophical approach, Warren and Zgourides advocate switching to discussing the probabilities versus the possibilities of such feared consequences occurring.[49]

Another method you can employ to tackle panic is to have your clients perform in-session voluntary hyperventilation as a means of reproducing panic symptoms and thereby learning to reattribute their symptoms to rapid breathing rather than catastrophic thinking. This technique is contraindicated in clients suffering from, for example, cardiac disease or severe asthma.[50] You can teach clients breathing retraining in order to bring their symptoms and themselves under greater control. Relaxation training can also be used to achieve greater control and as a form of distraction when clients are in a panic state '... because they are often incapable of Disputing well and of believing rational self-statements. We encourage them to use various kinds of distraction techniques [e.g. Yoga, meditation] to calm down and be unpanicked, and then to use Disputing and other RE[B]T methods.'[51]

You can encourage clients to expose themselves to avoided situations and activities in order to face their fears and test their catastrophic predictions, e.g. 'I'm going to disgrace myself in public and everyone will laugh at me'. In addition, they can learn to habituate themselves to the acute discomfort of their panic state – 'I can stand it but I don't like feeling this way' – and thereby develop high frustration tolerance (HFT). You may find it desirable to focus on and tackle your clients' secondary emotional problems, e.g. anxiety about anxiety or fear of fear, if you are to help them with their primary problems.

Ellis hypothesizes that the aforementioned secondary problems actually relate to the clients' anticipated discomfort in facing their fears or experiencing panic.[52] As usual, if you use REBT, you teach clients how to accept themselves with their panic disorder including, as in the above example, if they publicly 'disgrace' themselves and/or incur others' disapproval.

SUICIDAL CLIENTS

Suicidal ideas, plans or attempts are often part of the clinical picture of depression. Suicidal ideation can vary widely in its frequency, intensity and lethality: 'less severely suicidal individuals may report transient (1- to 2-minute), recurrent (once or twice a week) thoughts' while 'more severely suicidal individuals may have acquired materials (e.g. a rope or gun) to be used in the suicide attempt and may have established a location and time when they will be isolated from others so that they can accomplish the suicide'.[53] A sense of hopelessness about oneself and the future is one of the best predictors of suicide.[54] Fifteen per cent of severely depressed individuals eventually kill themselves.[55]

A study by Woods and Muller gave a general composite picture of the suicide-contemplator as someone '... who sees him/herself as a helpless victim of past and present circumstances who must nevertheless perform well, be approved of, and never have anything go wrong. Failure would be awful for it would prove one to be a worthless person.'[56] Reinecke suggests a two-stage process for tackling the suicidal client: managing the suicidal crisis and then longer-term treatment to identify and help change those factors which lead someone to contemplate suicide as a response option to adverse life events.[57]

During a suicidal crisis, Ellis states that '... I almost always directly confront their Irrational Beliefs – particularly their strongly held beliefs that the unfavourable conditions of their lives are *hopeless*, that they will *never* be able to change them, and that if they continue to live they will not be able to be happy *at all*'. Ellis emphasizes how in most cases he strongly and concretely disputes clients' suicidal ideas.[58]

Usually, you can isolate and tackle the immediate and key suicide-inducing beliefs (more general irrational ideas can wait until the crisis has moderated). Such beliefs and challenges may include:

Client: My family will be better off without me.
Therapist: How can you be so sure about this if you are dead?
Client: No one cares about me.
Therapist: If that's true, then why did your wife bring you to see me?
Client: I'll always be miserable, so why bother living?
Therapist: Your view of the future is coloured by your present depression. If I can help you to overcome this depression, will your view of the future remain the same?

You can point out to the client any in-session changes in thought, behaviour or mood as evidence that hope, no matter how slight, is returning.

McMullin suggests that in a severe crisis therapy should last several hours and instructs therapists to '... take no breaks. Flood the client with [cognitive] countering techniques; repeat them until the client comprehends their use' and '... present an assured, self-confident manner, to enhance the client's feelings of support'. Throughout the crisis, the client's reasons for killing himself should be challenged by the therapist's arguments for staying alive.[59]

Family, relatives and friends can be asked to keep a close watch on the client. However, if the home situation is one of the precipitants of the current crisis, hospitalization should be considered particularly if you actually believe that the client may kill himself. Sometimes you had better negotiate a contract with the client that he will contact you first before carrying out any suicidal plans. This gives you further opportunities to persuade the client to 'think again'. Once the crisis has passed and the client is relatively stable, longer-term therapy can focus on tackling the core irrational ideas that provide the breeding ground for his suicidal ideation, e.g. 'I have to be loved otherwise I'm utterly worthless'; 'I can't stand the humiliation and rejection every time I fail at something'.

Dealing with suicidal clients can be a highly stressful time for therapists, particularly if they subscribe to such irrational ideas as 'I absolutely must prevent him from killing himself to demonstrate my worth as a therapist'; 'I'm the only one who can save him'. Unless you identify and remove such ideas of your own if you have them, your clinical judgement is likely to be impaired and your desperation may well exacerbate an already tense situation.

WILFULLY RESISTANT CLIENTS

Wilfully resistant clients are those who deliberately and obstinately fight against therapy and frequently attempt to initiate and win power struggles with the therapist.[60] In an effort to make therapy more productive and less obstructive, you can offer to such clients the following points. Your own ego is not involved in therapy and therefore you will not be crestfallen if no progress is made or the client emerges 'victorious'. Thus you can say 'To be frank, I have no personal interest in whether or not your problems are sorted out but I will do my professional best to help you if you commit yourself to change'.

Unlike your own ego, the client's is usually on the line in power struggles and therefore she has to win in order not to see herself as a failure or worthless. There is no reason why she cannot behave in such a manner but she, not you, will continue to suffer from the psychological problems she avoids addressing if she resists therapy. Because your client may have abysmal LFT, she has not yet developed the capacity to face and endure the hard work associated with constructive change. Therefore she fritters away therapy time with her recalcitrant behaviour.

By persistently and forcefully disputing your client's beliefs, you may gain her cooperation and thereby both of you may achieve therapeutic change.

INVOLUNTARY CLIENTS

These are clients who reluctantly come to therapy at the insistence of others (e.g. parents, partners, courts, employers) and claim that they have no emotional or behavioural problems. Techniques that you can employ with such clients include the following.

1. Agreeing with clients that others are probably wrong about them but examining their claims anyway, e.g. 'I'm sure your wife does exaggerate how much you drink, but as we have this hour together shall we try and see why she's upset about it?'
2. Agreeing with clients that others probably have 'got it in for them' but that still does not solve their problems. For example, 'It must be very bad living at home with your parents on your case all the time, but your own behaviour is making life more difficult for you than it has to be'.
3. Agreeing with clients that therapy is probably a waste of time, and even though they have to be here they still retain the upper hand. Thus, 'I know you're here because attending therapy is part of the probation order but you still have the choice whether to cooperate or not. In that sense, you have more power than the courts or myself. So why not use that power in a way that might actually help you?'

Such methods may turn involuntary clients into voluntary ones and thereby induce them to engage constructively in therapy.

HIDDEN AGENDAS

Some of your clients may have real but hidden reasons why they enter therapy, rather than the ostensible ones they disclose to you. For example, a drug addict enters therapy 'to get off drugs for good' but actually seeks to sabotage it in order to prove he is a 'hopeless addict' and thereby continue his drug use. Or a woman attends couple counselling to save her relationship but, in reality, wants to end it but her guilt prevents her from doing so.

By giving all clients unconditional acceptance as fallible human beings, Ellis suggests that REBT can provide a therapeutic milieu which makes it more likely that clients will reveal their hidden agendas and undertake disputing of their associated irrational beliefs.[61] In the above examples, you can tackle the drug addict's hopelessness, 'I'll always be a junkie. I was probably born one.' And you can Dispute the woman's self-damnation, 'I would make him so miserable if I left him. I would be such a terrible person for doing that to him.' It is important that you remain alert for clues that might be offered by clients (e.g. the woman's frequently stated worries about her partner's inability to cope on his own rather than examining ways to save their faltering relationship) so that you reveal their real motives for being in therapy.

ARGUING

Clients may state, for example, that therapy will not be able to help them, that they will never change or that you do not understand 'real life' problems. Be cautious about arguing with clients over such issues because it may help to create a power struggle which results in an impasse in therapy. Dryden suggests saying something like this to your argumentative client: 'If you win the argument you also lose it because you will remain emotionally disturbed. If I win the argument you will also win because I can help you to overcome your emotional disturbance. Now whom do you want to win the argument?' Clients usually suggest you, the therapist, and then therapy can constructively proceed. If some clients state that they want to win they are likely to find they have achieved a Pyrrhic victory, i.e. won at considerable emotional cost to themselves (see section on wilfully resistant clients in this chapter).[62]

Some clients may wish to engage in a prolonged discussion of or argument over the use of the terms 'rational' and 'irrational'. As these terms are widely used in REBT, the impression might be created that the therapist has a superior understanding of these issues. Therefore the client might retort: 'Who can say what is rational and irrational? It's all subjective anyway.'

You should generally steer clear of philosophical debates on these issues. Point out their rather commonplace meanings in REBT, that is, rational means helping and irrational means defeating the client's chosen life goals and values. You will keep examining the client's subjective view of reality in order to determine and then help modify those aspects of it which are disturbance-producing and goal-blocking. You can assure your client that she will not be handed an 'objective reality kit' to assemble and then follow its instructions for a happier life.

If some of your clients persist in wanting to discuss the 'nature of reality', you can point out how time-consuming and ineffective it will prove to be. Thus, 'You might find such debate stimulating but it's hardly likely to overcome your procrastination and remove your guilt. Instead, let's discuss what steps are required to tackle your problems.' If some clients still resist, you can advise them to join a local debating society and come back to therapy when their philosophical focus is mainly on changing their self-defeating attitudes.

CONCLUSION

This chapter has shown how to address some clinical disorders, client groups and specific issues in counselling. It does not claim to be an authoritative or sufficient commentary on these problems and issues. For more comprehensive accounts, you can consult some relevant REBT and cognitive-behavioural therapy (CBT) handbooks and treatment manuals. However, if you are prepared to use on yourself as well as on your clients some of the strategies and techniques described in this chapter, you may find fewer blocks in therapy and may create a less stressful counselling environment in which you can practise.

NOTES

1. Ellis and Dryden, 1987; Young, 1988.
2. Ellis, 1985a, p. 1.

3. Ellis, 1985a.
4. Hauck, 1982, p. 60.
5. Ellis, 1985a.
6. Dryden, 1994a, p. 127.
7. Ellis, 1985a, p. 170.
8. Hauck, 1966.
9. Ellis, McInerney, DiGiuseppe and Yeager, 1988, p. 25.
10. Ellis, 1979d, 1980.
11. Greenwood, 1985, p. 224.
12. American Psychiatric Association, 1994, p. 424.
13. Warren and Zgourides, 1991, pp. 152–3.
14. Ellis, 1994b; Janoff-Bulman, 1985; Moore, 1993.
15. Muran and DiGiuseppe, 1994, p. 174.
16. Barlow, 1988.
17. Ellis, 1994c.
18. Warren and Zgourides, 1991.
19. Dryden, 1994b.
20. Warren and Zgourides, 1991, p. 129.
21. Ellis, 1994c, p. 132; see also 1994b.
22. Young and Lindemann, 1992, pp. 11–12, 23.
23. Beck, Freeman and Associates, 1990, p. 5.
24. Ellis, 1965, 1977b, 1983a, 1985a, 1994d.
25. American Psychiatric Association, 1994, p. 654.
26. Ellis, 1994d.
27. Ellis, 1985a, 1994d.
28. Leaf and DiGiuseppe, 1992, p. 105.
29. Ellis, 1985a, p. 144.
30. Ellis, 1994d, p. 111.
31. Ellis, 1994d, p. 109.
32. Bresler, 1988; American Psychiatric Association, 1994.
33. American Psychiatric Association, 1994, p. 539.
34. Fairburn and Cooper, 1989, p. 277.
35. Ellis, 1990c.
36. Fairburn and Cooper, 1989, p. 307.
37. Bresler, 1988.
38. McCrea, 1991.
39. Fairburn and Cooper, 1989, p. 300.
40. Bresler, 1988, p. 14.
41. American Psychiatric Association, 1994, p. 545.
42. Fairburn, 1995.
43. Woods and Grieger, 1993.
44. Dryden, 1989.
45. American Psychiatric Association, 1994, p. 397.
46. Salkovskis and Clark, 1991, p. 216.
47. Dryden, 1989.
48. Dryden, 1989, p. 62.
49. Warren and Zgourides, 1991.

50. Clark, 1989.
51. Ellis, quoted in Dryden, 1991, p. 68.
52. Ellis, 1979d, 1980d.
53. American Psychiatric Association, 1994, p. 322.
54. Beck, Steer, Kovacs and Garrison, 1985.
55. Reported in Fennell, 1989.
56. Woods and Muller, 1988.
57. Reinecke, 1994.
58. Ellis, 1987d, p. 135.
59. McMullin, 1986, p. 270.
60. Ellis, 1985a.
61. Ellis, 1985a.
62. Dryden, in Dryden and Neenan, 1995.

CHAPTER 9

Occupational Stress and Group Work

Because REBT is a psychoeducational approach, it very easily adapts to a variety of arenas. Although the majority of REBT counsellors use this approach with clients in individual counselling, it can also be used in group therapy, family and couples counselling, weekend marathons, seminars or in industrial training settings.[1] In this chapter we will be focusing on two specific areas which can be particularly time–efficient and cost-effective: industrial stress management training and group stress counselling. As many REBT counsellors see clients suffering from occupational stress, we will first cover the main organizational and occupational stressors and then consider industrial stress management training and group stress counselling. We will also cover pre-training material and suitable bibliotherapy.

We would recommend that you become experienced in using REBT with individual clients before attempting to run stress counselling or training groups. In addition, if you are not experienced in working with groups, it is advisable to either receive specific training in group work or, initially, run a group with an experienced group leader. One of the main reasons that we make this recommendation is that the dynamics of interaction and communication patterns are more complex in groups than in individual stress counselling. Therefore the counsellor requires additional skills. For example, assertiveness skills are needed to deal with compulsive talkers or disruptive individuals.

UNDERSTANDING ORGANIZATIONAL AND OCCUPATIONAL STRESS

It has been estimated that in the United Kingdom, 360 million working days are lost every year through sickness.[2] This costs industry £8 billion approximately per annum. At least 50 per cent of the lost days are stress related, according to the Health and Safety Executive, while in the USA it is estimated that executives are costing their companies $20 billion per annum as a result of stress-related illnesses. According to statistics stress has become one of the major causes of absenteeism in the workplace. The personal cost of prolonged stress to individuals is the negative effect it has on their health and well-being. Prolonged stress can lead to early death due to coronary heart disease (CHD) or other life threatening disorders (see Chapter 1). The main symptoms of organizational stress are high absenteeism, high staff turnover, increased health care claims, increased industrial accidents, industrial relations difficulties, lowered efficiency, low morale, poor quality control, poor job performance, staff burnout and suicide.

Although each occupation has its own potential stressors, there are some common factors:[3]

- home/work interface;
- internal demands (i.e. Irrational Beliefs);
- factors intrinsic to the job;
- organizational structure and climate;
- career development;
- role in the organization;
- relationships at work.

Figure 9.1 illustrates the relationship between the common factors, the individual, the home/work interface and the symptoms. These issues will now be considered along with interventions you can use to deal with these problems. Possible organizational interventions will be covered too.

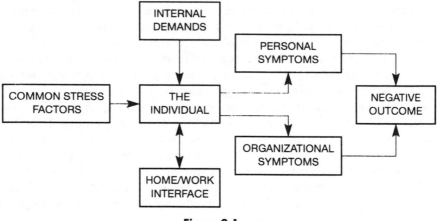

Figure 9.1

Home/work interface

If individuals are distressed due to problems at work then this can affect their home life and vice versa. A typical example would be an employee who is having to deal with the emotional and practical problems of a close family bereavement. Understandably, this stress scenario is likely to reduce his or her performance at work, which subsequently may even lead to disciplinary action by management. Unfortunately this can exacerbate an already difficult home life. However, if the cause of the reduced performance is recognized by management or the occupational health department at an early stage, then the employee could be referred to a confidential stress counselling service or in-house counsellor to help come to terms with the bereavement and also receive practical advice about associated problems such as probate, etc.[4] Large organizations may be able to afford to employ a counsellor, whereas smaller organizations may need to use either an Employee Assistance Programme or an external counsellor.

Internal demands

As illustrated in the previous chapters, individuals usually distress themselves by placing absolutist and dogmatic demands upon themselves, others and the world. The workplace is no exception. In our clinical and occupational experience it is not just an external pressure or stressor, such as a deadline, that causes occupational stress but internal demands or pressures individuals make upon themselves. Palmer highlighted a number of internal demands or Irrational Beliefs that can be the major contributory factor to occupational stress:[5]

- I/others must perform well at all times otherwise it would be awful;
- I/others must always reach deadlines;
- I/others must be perfect;
- The organization must treat me fairly at all times;
- I absolutely should get what I want otherwise I can't stand it;
- Significant others must appreciate my work otherwise I am worthless.

If you follow REBT, you can use disputes and interventions described in the previous chapters to help stressed employees change their dysfunctional thinking for more effective and less disturbing thinking. In our experience, rigid perfectionist beliefs are one of the major contributory factors to occupational stress.

Factors intrinsic to the job

Many differing stressors intrinsic to the job can cause stress. Some of the more common environmental workplace stressors are:

- air pollution
- fibres/dust
- heat
- humidity
- lighting
- nicotine
- noise
- noxious chemicals
- 'sick building' syndrome
- static electricity
- uncomfortable chairs/work stations
- VDU screen glare.

These stressors can cause a wide range of different physical ailments including allergic reactions, backache, chest infections, deafness, eye strain, headache, neckache and skin rashes. Not surprisingly, an employee's general morale and work productivity can also be affected. Therefore, you can assess whether environmental stressors are a factor that may be directly causing the client's physical symptoms of stress. You can also undertake a behavioural analysis to ascertain exactly what the client was doing before the stress-related symptoms developed. A typical transcript of a REBT stress counselling session, in which the counsellor is attempting to discover the cause of a recurrent neckache, is as follows:

> Counsellor: Does there appear to be any pattern to when your neckache occurs?
> Client: No. It seems to come and go.
> Counsellor: It may be helpful if we look at a specific example to help us ascertain the possible causes of your neckache. Think back to the last time you had neckache. Can you remember?

(The counsellor wishes to examine a specific example to assess whether the neckaches occur at random.)

> Client: Yes. It was last Monday and I was at work. I had it by late afternoon.
> Counsellor: Were you doing anything different than usual that day?

(The counsellor is checking whether he did anything different from his usual routine that may be the cause of the neckaches.)

> Client: No. It was a typical Monday. You know, the usual thing; plenty of telephone calls and arranging meetings for the week.
> Counsellor: Tell me exactly what you did once you arrived at work.
> Client: I sat down and opened my mail. I had a fair amount to deal with, as it was a typical Monday. I then listened to my answerphone and collected my faxes from John's office. Then it was my coffee break.
> Counsellor: Then ...
> Client: It was about 11.00 a.m. I spent the rest of the morning on the telephone. I had a quick lunch as I was so busy. Then I spent until my afternoon coffee break talking to customers on the telephone about difficulties they had encountered with the new computer programme.
> Counsellor: So when did you first notice that your neck was aching?
> Client: Hmmm. By the time I was having my afternoon break. Thinking about it, I reckon that I generally get my neckache at the beginning of the week.
> Counsellor: And Monday usually involves a day on the telephone.
> Client: Yes.
> Counsellor: How exactly do you hold your telephone handset?

(In the counsellor's experience, some individuals may give themselves either tension neckaches or headaches because of the way they hold a telephone handset.)

> Client: Like this. Between my ear and shoulder.

(Client shows the counsellor how he usually holds the handset between his ear and shoulder.)

Counsellor: Hmmm. I suspect that you may find that the cause of your neckache is spending the day on the telephone and holding the handset in such an awkward position. To see if my hypothesis is correct, I suggest that next Monday when you are at work you sit upright in your chair, keeping your neck upright without using your shoulders to conveniently position your handset. Perhaps try and stagger your calls during the day, giving yourself short breaks. What do you think?

Client: I must admit, it does make sense. In fact, it is usually days I'm in the office when I get neckache and not when I'm out on the road visiting customers.

In this example, if the counsellor initially assumed that the cause of the neckache was due to Irrational Beliefs about the customers and did not first undertake a systematic behavioural analysis then it is likely that this client would not have found a main cause of his problem. It is highly recommended that counsellors use hypothesis testing to ensure that they have discovered the main cause of a problem, especially if ergonomics are involved, i.e. the relationship between workers and their environment – in particular, the machines and equipment they use. Referral to other health professionals may be desirable in some circumstances.

Other stressful factors intrinsic to the job that REBT stress counsellors can explore with clients or trainees attending a stress management workshop are:

- boring repetitive tasks
- dangerous work
- deadlines
- excessive travel
- isolated working conditions
- long hours
- shift work
- work underload/overload
- work too difficult for the individual.

However, the REBT stress counsellor would also investigate whether the client held Irrational Beliefs about these possible stress scenarios which would help to exacerbate the person's stress reaction.

A number of surveys indicate that time pressures and deadlines are perceived as major stressors by executives. In Britain, the amount of travel associated with work is also considered to be a problem, although more recently there is an increasing concern about possible redundancy and unemployment. Research has found that some occupations are more stressful than others. For example, acting, advertising, building, dentistry, journalism, mining, the police force, the prison service, are more stressful than accountancy, astronomy, biochemistry, geology, insurance, the Church, nature conservancy and horticulture.[6]

Organizational structure and climate

In many companies the organizational structure and climate may limit the autonomy of the employee. Workers may believe, quite correctly, that they have little influence or control over their workload. This can contribute to apathy, job dissatisfaction, reduced self-esteem, resentment and a loss of identity. This tends to increase rates of absenteeism. However, as self-esteem is dependent upon an individual's belief system REBT stress counsellors and trainers would focus their intervention on improving self-acceptance (see Chapter 2). Organizations wishing to alleviate these problems can increase participation in decision-making and team work to help over-come an actual or perceived lack of control. Where appropriate, trade unions can be involved in planning job rotation and employees could elect their own supervisors. This can help to increase job morale and commitment to the work.

Due to the recent recession many organizations have either made or are consider-ing making redundancies. Employees living under this threat can suffer from increased levels of stress. Possibly the only way to help deal with this problem is to ensure that the senior management communicate as quickly as possible on all issues. If a company has a history of making last-minute announcements then employees are likely to be less trusting. REBT stress counsellors would focus on two levels with clients working under these conditions.

Initially, the counsellor would target the client's Irrational Beliefs relating to the current or feared problem for disputation. This is particularly important if the client is feeling depressed about the situation and is unable to cope. In addition practical problem-solving would be focused on improving the situation, for example, teaching a non-assertive client assertion skills and coping imagery exercises to help him or her ask the employer relevant questions.

When it is likely that the client may lose their job then other practical interven-tions are employed such as job seeking, up-dating the client's CV or résumé, and referral to a careers adviser. Some companies engage stress management trainers to run courses to help their staff deal with the stress of losing their jobs. Assuming the employees wish to attend these courses, we have found that teaching them the ABCDE paradigm of REBT has proved very helpful. In large organizations, such as government bodies, we have found that teaching the ABCDE paradigm as part of a seminar on 'Coping with redundancy' is a useful additional skill for many staff. These groups can be cost-effective as many employees can attend each seminar. Practical suggestions on coping with redundancy or lay-offs are also included.

The recent economic recession has triggered changes in industry. Reduced staffing levels, the increased use of technology and job relocations are life changes or events that can contribute to stress in employees. Retraining, outplacement coun-selling and change management seminars or workshops may help to reduce the negative effects of these types of change.

Ageism, sexism and racism can also be prevalent in some organizations. Employers can draw up a set policy and procedure to deal with these areas. Employers should be seen to be proactive as well as just reactive. The policy needs to be displayed on notice boards and enforced whenever necessary.

Career development

For many employees career development is an important issue. Unfortunately, promotion prospects can become increasingly limited at higher levels of the organi-zation. For some individuals the only apparent solution to this problem is to change jobs. It is now more commonplace for older employees to regularly receive training to enable them to use new technology. Employees can become stressed and anxious about these and other challenges such as learning new management skills. Also research has found that older employees tend to be anxious about redundancy (lay-offs), demotion, obsolescence, lack of job security and forced early retirement. These issues can often trigger underlying Irrational Beliefs or schemata that are associated with self-esteem and self-worth and can lead to depression. REBT counsellors or trainers would focus their interventions at disputing these Irrational Beliefs and at developing coping strategies.

Role in the organization

Research shows that different roles in an organization can lead to varying amounts of stress, although this can depend upon the person–job fit. Generally, employees who are responsible for subordinates are more likely to suffer from coronary heart disease than those who are responsible for machinery. There are a number of different role demands that can contribute to stress, i.e. ambiguity, conflict, definition, expectations, incompatibility, overload and underload. It is worth noting that many employees do not recognize these external sources of their stress. We will briefly consider the role demands that we have found as major contributory factors to stress in employees.

Role ambiguity occurs when employees are unsure about the role expectations that are required of them. They may have unclear role objectives, and may have received conflicting or inadequate information about their job. In these cases they will seldom know what behaviours will lead to a fulfilment of the role expectations. Induction training and a clear written contract may help to clarify the position for new employees and others with whom they work.

Role conflict involves different role expectations made by the following groups on the employee:

- superiors
- superiors' superior
- peers
- clients
- subordinates
- subordinates' subordinates.

The employee may also have expectations that differ from her or his employment contract. One form of conflict occurs when the employee's own value system conflicts with the expectations of the organization; for example, in a recession a vegetarian may work for a restaurant serving meat dishes. Other forms of conflict may occur where the expected role behaviour is too difficult to perform or too many different roles are expected for the particular employee.

Employees can also become stressed about role overload as they experience difficulty coping with their work. Conversely, with role underload employees may not feel challenged and they may become bored. Each job needs to be assessed to avoid both role overload or underload. Although the other forms of role demands may be difficult for employees to recognize, most realize when they are doing too much work.

REBT stress counsellors and trainers can help clients recognize the specific role demands that may be contributing to their occupational stress and develop strategies to attempt to overcome them. In many cases, employees need to use assertion and communication skills to discuss their specific role demand problems with their managers. In addition the counsellor or trainer usually needs to examine and dispute any Irrational Beliefs the employee holds about these particular problems. It is worth noting that in our experience the Irrational Belief 'I must not lose control, otherwise it would be awful' is often present with clients who are stressed about role overload, role conflict and role ambiguity. Irrational Beliefs involving low self-worth and low frustration tolerance may also be present.

Relationships at work

Interpersonal relationships are one of the main causes of stress in both large and small organizations. Quick and Quick have found a number of specific interpersonal stressors that can be a source of occupational stress including abrasive personalities, peer/group pressures, leadership style, social density and social incongruence.[7] If staff, or in particular managers, act aggressively they often benefit from assertion skills training. In addition, key staff can receive training in human resources skills such as listening and communication. Unhelpful passive-aggressive behaviours include:

- inappropriate anger/hostility;
- aggressive body posture;
- pointing finger;
- angry intonation;
- verbal put-downs, e.g. 'you'd better', 'come on', 'you should', 'you must';
- sulking.

Employees who act in a hostile or bullying manner usually cause interpersonal difficulties in the workplace. As these individuals are usually Type A too (i.e. aggressive, pressured by time constraints, talk/walk/eat quickly, ambitious) they unwittingly increase their chances of dying early from coronary heart disease.[8] Although assertion training can be useful in these cases, in our clinical experience with extreme Type A individuals in-depth REBT counselling is required too. Short stress management courses are usually insufficient as extremely low frustration tolerance and low self-esteem are normally present.

Relationships between co-workers can be negative due to rivalry, competition and 'office politics', yet they can also provide a social support structure which helps to buffer individuals from stress.[9] Social support networks are sometimes unintentionally created when organizations offer their employees sports and social facilities.[10] For some employees, the first time they start to share their problems with each other and gain mutual support is while attending a stress management training workshop. When running these workshops, the trainer needs to ensure that time is set aside for employees to discuss and share workplace problems.

INDUSTRIAL STRESS MANAGEMENT INTERVENTIONS

We have now considered a number of the issues involved with organizational and occupational stress. Although we have already indicated the type of interventions organizations, REBT stress counsellors or REBT stress management trainers/consultants can undertake, we will briefly cover some of the other issues involved and make a number of recommendations.

Industrial interventions can be made at three different levels:[11]

Level	Intervention
Primary:	Remove hazard or reduce employees' exposure to it, or its impact on them.
Secondary:	Improve the organization's ability to recognize and deal with stress-related problems as they occur.
Tertiary:	Help employees cope with and recover from work-related problems.

REBT-based stress management interventions that focus on the employees' appraisal of potential stressors are useful at all three intervention levels. At the primary level, REBT stress management training can help to reduce the impact of stressors upon the employee. At the secondary level, it can help managers and key staff to recognize stress in their employees. At the tertiary level, REBT stress counselling or group training can help employees cope with and recover from work-related problems such as burnout. One of the goals of REBT training in industry would be to prevent employees from becoming stressed in the first place and to be able to recognize the source of stress – i.e. is it from external or internal pressures, or a combination of both? – and then finally deal with the stressor.[12] Unfortunately, straightforward solutions seldom exist for the reduction or alleviation of organizational and occupational stressors. Usually there is a short-term financial cost for a company if an effective intervention is going to be made. However, the long-term gains in production and reduced absenteeism may well be worth the initial cost.

Undertaking a Stress Audit which focuses on how stressed staff are feeling and from where they perceive the workplace pressures to be emanating, is usually a good starting point before any stress management intervention is undertaken.[13] Once an intervention(s) has been chosen it will need to be assessed and evaluated in a systematic manner to ensure that the intervention actually helped the organization and its staff.[14] All too often a stress management workshop is seen as the panacea when in fact it could raise more issues than it resolves. The Stress Audit may indicate that an Employee Assistance Programme or a stress counselling service could be more effective in the long run.[15] We have found the computerized version of the Occupational Stress Indicator (OSI) useful for Stress Audits and also invaluable for stress counselling and stress management workshops.[16] It provides individual reports and profiles for employees and the organization, and indicates changes both the individual and the organization can make to reduce stress. It can also be used as an evaluation tool to assess the effectiveness of an intervention.

Some interventions which involve workplace change can lead to increased levels of stress if they are not implemented properly. Annual Stress Audits involving employee participation may help to keep the subject of stress and its management alive and on the agenda. It can also form part of a Total Quality Management programme. It is recommended that employees from different parts of the organization are included on a stress 'working party' as active participation may be necessary for the employees to take the process seriously. In some organizations that have a 'macho' culture, initially it is preferable to talk about 'managing pressure' as stress may be seen as a weakness that 'must not be admitted' publicly. If this is not dealt with in a sensitive manner then employees may be resistant about attending stress management workshops.

In the next section we focus on the content of industrial stress management workshops.

Industrial stress management workshops and courses

Assuming a particular organization has identified a need for a stress management workshop or course, an experienced REBT stress counsellor or trainer may be employed to provide the training. An in-house REBT counsellor would be in an ideal position to offer employees suitable training. The duration of the workshop usually depends upon time and financial restraints. The workshop could last between one and five days, or consist of ongoing weekly sessions lasting between one and four hours for between five and ten sessions. We have found that, for convenience, organizations tend to prefer one- or two-day courses as this is easier to organize than ongoing short sessions.

The participants of an industrial stress management training group tend to differ from clients attending stress counselling groups as the former may not necessarily be currently suffering from stress and are sometimes just attending to learn how to prevent or manage stress. In stress counselling or therapy groups, clients are normally suffering from the effects of stress and are usually interested in learning how to cope or manage current problems and this will often lead to self-disclosure of an intimate nature.[17] Therefore the needs of each group tend to differ and REBT stress counsellors should take this into account when working in different settings.

Employees attending training courses at work usually receive an educational format whereby the trainer teaches them relevant theory and they may practise specific skills such as sales techniques or assertion. Due to the active, directive, versatile and systematic nature of the REBT approach it can also be taught in a similar fashion. This avoids any similarity with therapy which is generally less acceptable to employees in workplace settings. Prospective workshop participants can be asked to complete a brief questionnaire or be interviewed to discover what they would like to learn from the stress management workshop prior to attending the course. Once this is known, participants can be set relevant pre-course reading or self-help guides to read or complete which focus on the nature and consequences of stress, and the cognitive dynamics of stress including the disputation of Irrational Beliefs.[18] To help participants become more aware of their workplace stressors, they are usually asked to keep a 'Stress Diary' for one workday. This involves keeping a note of the day's events, in particular situations that they become stressed about. They are asked to bring their diary to the course for later discussion.

In stress management workshops, apart from coffee breaks, for maximum effectiveness all of the time available is focused on stress and its management. Typical course or workshop contents for a two-day 'stress management' or 'managing pressure to improve performance' programme are below (adapted from Palmer).[19]

COURSE CONTENTS

1. Discussion of ground rules (including discussing the benefits of confidentiality, if unclear to the participants).
2. Ask what the participants are hoping to learn and achieve over the duration of the course. (This confirms their requirements they sent in prior to the course.)
3. Participants share their 'Stress Diaries' with the group if they so wish. The trainer focuses on how different members of the group would have felt and dealt with the disclosed stress scenarios emphasizing the diverse cognitive, emotive and behavioural dynamics; in particular, highlighting one person's stress as another person's challenge or pleasure.
4. Discussion of a simple definition of stress e.g. too much or too little pressure leads to stress; pressure can be internal or external, or a combination of both. (Include 'demands' versus 'coping resources' if helpful.)
5. Small group work to consider the symptoms of stress.
6. Group debrief.
7. Discuss the psychophysiology of stress. (If available, use suitable video that explains the physiology of stress in simple terms.)
8. Participants use biodots (i.e. biofeedback instruments) to monitor skin temperature. Explain that a relaxed state leads to vasodilation.
9. Teach the ABCDE paradigm. Illustrate how Irrational Beliefs and twisted thinking (cognitive distortions) exacerbate stress.
10. Thinking skills practice, i.e. in small group work, participants discuss a recent stress scenario and help each other to challenge Irrational Beliefs and major cognitive distortions (in p.m. of first day of course). (See also Appendices 9 and 10 below, pages 193–4.)
11. Participants can be shown how to use an ABCDE form to aid practice of the thinking skills (see Box 9.1 and Appendix 5). Small group work focusing on current problem using the ABCDE form (in a.m. of second day).
12. Teach a method of relaxation to the group (see Chapter 6).
13. If available, the trainer demonstrates how to use a Galvanic Skin Response (GSR) biofeedback instrument to monitor the effectiveness of the relaxation exercise. Then the trainer shows the group how quickly a person can trigger the stress response just by thinking of a stressful situation. (This highlights how the situation itself does not cause stress but it is the individual's beliefs about it that trigger the stress response.) If sufficient GSR instruments are available, each participant can practise relaxing by using the GSR as a monitor.
14. Imagery techniques can be taught to the group; for example, rational-emotive imagery, coping and time-projection imagery (see Chapter 6).[20]
15. Lifestyle interventions such as nutrition, weight/alcohol control, exercise, stopping smoking, time management, assertion can be discussed depending upon the needs and interests of the group.
16. Group discussion on organizational/occupational stress. Possible workplace interventions discussed in small group work.
17. Type A behaviour, locus of control and workplace coping strategies discussed.[21]
18. Group OSI reports given to each participant. The trainer explains each section of the report and leads discussion about the issues raised. (NB: Although useful, it is not essential to use an OSI in the workshop. This also applies to activity 19.)

Box 9.1 An ABCDE form

Activating Workplace Problem (A)	Self-Defeating Beliefs (B)	Emotional/Behavioural Consequences (C)	Disputing Self-Defeating Beliefs (D)	New Effective Approach to Problem (E)
Project deadline	I must reach the dead-line	Very anxious; irritable with work colleagues	Logical: Just because I want to reach the dead-line how does it logically follow that I must reach it?	Although it's strongly preferable to reach the deadline, logically I don't have to.
May not reach the dead-line	If I don't it will be awful and I would be a total failure		Empirical: Where is the evidence that my demand must be granted?	There is no evidence that I will get what I demand even if it is preferable.
			Am I being realistic? If I don't reach the deadline will the outcome be awful and would I become a total failure?	If I don't reach the deadline, the outcome may be bad but hardly a horror and it would not prove that I was a total failure.
			Pragmatic: Where is it getting me holding on to this belief?	As long as I hold on to this belief I will remain very anxious and waste my time worrying instead of working constructively on the project.
				If I change my attitude I will feel very concerned but remain problem-focused and more likely to reach the deadline. If I don't reach the dead-line, I will not beat myself up.

Box 9.2 *Stress management plan*

DATE: 12/1/96

ACTION TO BE TAKEN BY: EMMA

Thinking Skills:	Dispute the demands I place upon myself, in particular, my perfectionist musturbatory beliefs.
	Whenever I become stressed about a situation, remind myself that things may be bad, but seldom, if ever, awful!
Imagery:	Practise rational-emotive imagery when I am stressed about future events.
	Practise coping imagery before each presentation to the board of directors.
Time Management:	At work, start the day by making a 'to do' list; and keep to it.
Assertion:	Be less passive-aggressive with my work colleagues. Say 'No', when I need to.
	Instead of arguing with my boss, use workable compromise instead.
Relaxation:	Ensure that I make time for my daily relaxation exercise. Remember to breathe slowly from my stomach whenever I become stressed.
Nutrition:	Eat less fatty food; eat fresh fruit daily. Eat fish at least twice per week. Reduce coffee intake and drink herbal tea instead.

---

19. Individual OSI reports given to each participant. Trainer answers general questions about the reports and highlights that the 'logical thinking' section relates to how effectively the individual is using thinking skills.
20a Small group work focusing on each participant's workplace problems and also on how they can overcome these issues. For example, if appropriate, start to act assertively with a passive-aggressive manager, and only feel concerned instead of feeling anxious about this exercise.
20b During activity 20a, the trainer can discuss the individual OSI reports with each participant that needs further feedback or guidance.
21. Debrief activity 20a. If appropriate, a group stress management plan is developed. For example, how the group can manage their manager's excessive demands.

22. Individual stress management plans developed by each participant (see Box 9.2) and then discussion in small groups on how to ensure that they can keep to their plans and overcome any obstacles that may arise.
23. Discussion of 'where to go from here'.
24. Possibility of follow-up day discussed if appropriate, and if acceptable to the organization.

The course content is flexible and may depend upon what the participants wish to cover as long as the focus is directed at understanding stress and learning stress management skills. A one- or half-day workshop can still include an explanation of the basic psychophysiology, the ABCDE paradigm and other helpful strategies and techniques. Although courses can concentrate solely on teaching the ABCDEs of REBT, a comprehensive and holistic approach is likely to benefit more participants even if palliative techniques and strategies, such as relaxation, are taught especially if participants are suffering from chronic problems (i.e. not of recent onset). Employees cannot usually be excluded from attending stress management workshops just because they do not conceptualize stress in the REBT model of psychological problems. In fact, some research shows that workshop participants can benefit from talking to each other about stress without necessarily being taught any stress management skills by a trainer.

Participants 'feel better' (as Ellis shows) because of the supportive and/or cathartic effect of sharing personal experiences. However, in our experience, an important part of relapse prevention is allowing participants to anticipate future stress scenarios and decide how to deal with them by planning, and practising strategies or techniques learnt during the workshop. This is not possible if participants have not been taught new strategies. One of the aims of a REBT stress management workshop is for the participants to 'do better' rather than just 'feel better', subsequently becoming their own effective stress managers and this usually requires adequate preparation.[22]

A one-day or half-day follow-up would focus on how the participants fared with the application of the strategies and techniques. Often an important issue is how they have prevented themselves from regularly practising the techniques and strategies that formed part of their individual stress management action plans. Strategies and techniques would be discussed and demonstrated again, if necessary, and new techniques introduced if appropriate.[23] This will help employees 'stay better'.

Some organizations will allow a course to run over a period of weeks. Kushnir and Malkinson found that the course contents below helped a non-clinical group of industrial workers to reduce cognitive weariness, Irrational Beliefs and somatic complaints even at long-term follow-up after 20 months.[24]

COURSE CONTENTS

1. Introduction of the ABC model of REBT.
2. Identification of Irrational and Rational Beliefs and their emotional and behavioural consequences.
3. Explaining and elaborating the concepts of stress and burnout.
4. Analysing personal experiences of stress and burnout in terms of the ABC model.
5. Disputation of Irrational Beliefs and changing them into rational ones.

6. Assertiveness training which focused on the interaction with superiors. (This was a major concern of many of the participants.)
7. Vignettes. This was one of the main teaching techniques used throughout the course. Realistic interpersonal exchanges at work with superiors and co-workers were presented and analysed in terms of REBT principles.
8. Relaxation. Each meeting was terminated with a five-minute muscle relaxation session.
9. Homework. Participants were assigned homework according to specific topics dealt with at the meeting.

The workshop was preceded by a preliminary two-hour lecture on stress management and exhaustion, which outlined the causes of workplace stress and a variety of coping techniques. The workshop started one week later. Five weekly meetings were held, each lasting four hours. The results of this study highlight how REBT can help individuals not only to 'feel better' but, more importantly, 'do and stay better' too. Interestingly, the results of the long-term follow-up indicated that a booster session focusing on additional assertiveness skills training would have been beneficial, whereas there was less need for more rationality training.

Rational Effectiveness Training

Ellis and DiMattia are keen advocates of Rational Effectiveness Training which is a method of teaching basic principles of interpersonal relations to groups of individuals and is particularly applicable to all levels of management, and to others who work in the area of 'people contact'.[25] It helps staff to deal with interpersonal stressors by coaching them in REBT skills (see previous chapters). In this section we will consider the goals of the training and the approach of the group leader.

The Rational Effectiveness Training goals are:[26]

(a) achieving more through eliminating fear of failure;
(b) becoming tolerant and less hostile towards superiors, associates, subordinates;
(c) gaining unqualified self-acceptance and self-respect;
(d) achieving minimal anxiety and insecurity;
(e) gaining maximum self-determination;
(f) achieving high frustration tolerance;
(g) unchaining the influence of the past;
(h) acquiring vitally absorbing interests.

In REBT stress management training and rational effectiveness training the group leader uses a number of strategies. The leader:

1. directly gets things moving by bringing up a specific kind of problem and urging one of the members of the group to speak up about it;
2. does not hesitate to give his or her authoritative analysis of what participants are doing to needlessly disturb themselves. The leader encourages other group members to give their interpretations of how their colleagues manage to upset themselves;

3. ensures that the discussion avoids abstractions and generalizations, and focuses on real problems in concrete terms;
4. actively steers participants towards a deeper understanding of problems in REBT terms;
5. will calmly but definitely take sides at various points: e.g. tactfully to correct a group member while upholding another member;
6. formulates a hypothesis about a group member's problem and discusses it with the group, demonstrating how thinking more rationally may lead to better results. Before the discussion has ended the leader will ensure that the group member understands clearly how to apply what has been covered in the discussion to his or her own specific job problem;
7. draws into the discussion some of the weaker members of the group so that they too will understand what is being discussed and will have a maximum chance to change some of their own irrational or non-rational views;
8. summarizes some of the salient aspects of a discussion so that they will be more applicable to other members of the group;
9. is catalytic and didactic throughout the session, continually encouraging the participants to be self-ventilating and helpful to themselves as well as to the other group members. The leader is both a *discussion* leader and a discussion *leader*. The leader is teacher of rational viewpoints as well as teaching in a Socratic manner that maximally involves the other group members and encourages them to think things out for themselves;
10. is highly authoritative without being in the least authoritarian and therefore combines the best features of democratic participation and open-ended enquiry;
11. focuses the group on a specific topic ensuring that all of the members devote their attention to that topic rather than engaging in small talk;
12. suggests homework assignments and supplementary reading;
13. makes an effort to see that some kind of closure occurs for each participant as a result of the training session.

This approach is suited to the hard world of business and industry as it remains problem focused and helps employees to maximize their performance and reduce interpersonal stressors. In the next section we focus on group stress counselling.

Group stress counselling

Normally group stress counselling differs from group stress management training in that the former is generally more psychotherapeutic in its approach and is mainly used in counselling or clinical settings. Yet as the REBT approach is psychoeducational and the counsellor is systematic and active-directive in both counselling and training arenas these subtleties can be considered as largely irrelevant. One of the important distinguishing factors is that members of stress counselling groups are usually suffering from stress when they first join and often they have been referred to the group by health professionals. This is in contrast to participants of stress management training groups who may not be suffering from stress and are usually interested in learning about stress and preventive stress management techniques. Also stress management training tends to include more formal educational input. However, there are no hard and fast rules.

We are keen advocates of group stress counselling as it has many advantages. Some of the key advantages are listed below:

1. Probably one of the most important advantages is that groups are cost-effective as the counsellor can see many clients.[27] The ABCDE paradigm and stress management techniques can be demonstrated to a number of individuals simultaneously thus saving time.
2. In group stress counselling, several group members can challenge an individual's Irrational Beliefs. This has the secondary benefit of powerfully reinforcing Rational Beliefs for the group members. By helping others, group members learn to help themselves. We agree with Lazarus who believes that 'consensual validation tends to carry more weight than the views of one person, even if that person is a highly respected authority'.[28]
3. Individuals quickly realize that they are not alone in suffering from particular problems. This reinforces the concept of human fallibility, encourages self-acceptance, provides reassuring information about the non-uniqueness of their problems, subsequently reducing stress that arises from Irrational Beliefs about uncertainty.[29]
4. The group member is frequently offered a wider range of possible solutions to problems than would normally be offered in individual counselling.
5. By listening to other members' problems, an individual can become aware of solutions to difficulties that he or she has not already encountered in life. This would have a preventive function and could be an important long-term benefit of group work.
6. As individuals start to improve, this reinforces other group members' belief in the approach as effective and also gives them hope that they too can change.
7. Interpersonal or social skills deficits are more easily dealt with in group settings, as individuals can practise with each other new skills under the guidance of the counsellor.
8. Group members can use peer pressure to encourage members to undertake homework assignments.
9. The group provides a setting for risk-attacking and shame-attacking exercises in a relatively safe environment.
10. Members can learn useful stress management skills from each other as well as from the counsellor.
11. Revealing problems to the group may be in itself therapeutic for the individual. Gradually the individual starts to learn that self-disclosure is not as shameful as he or she had previously first thought.
12. Group stress counselling tends to provide a more stimulating and more activating kind of involvement than individual treatment often does.[30]
13. Group members can offer each other support in times of crisis.

Although there are many advantages of group stress counselling, Ellis has noted that there are a number of intrinsic disadvantages when compared to other therapy settings. These include members unintentionally misleading other members or formulating poor solutions to problems. Instead of providing challenging homework exercises they suggest overwhelming exercises. They can allow a member, if the counsellor does not intervene, to get away with minimal participation and hence minimal change.[31] We will now look at how stress counselling groups are run and the type of exercises or techniques the counsellor is likely to use.

In non-industrial settings, such as adult education institutions, colleges, thera-peutic communities, hospitals, training and counselling centres, REBT stress management groups can be run in a similar manner to those described in the previ-ous sections. The educational format used in industrial settings suits both adolescents and adults and for many people is less threatening than joining a stress counselling or therapy group. Obviously, occupational issues may be left out of a programme depending upon the members of the group.

As with stress management training groups, stress counselling groups also have a variety of formats. We will briefly consider the options.

(a) Ongoing groups which meet weekly for between one and a half and two and a half hours. These groups can be open-ended and participants can join when there is an available space. Or the group can be run for a fixed period of time. This is generally between six and twelve sessions, with a follow-up session a month or two later.

(b) One- or two-day stress counselling groups can be run lasting about eight hours per day.

(c) Stress counselling group marathon sessions can be run for up to fourteen straight hours with from ten to sixteen participants.

The format adopted will usually depend upon the setting in which the counsellor is working. Counsellors working in hospitals or in general practice tend to run open-ended or closed groups on a weekly or twice weekly basis, whereas counsellors working in private practice often find it easier to set up one- or two-day events. However, one- or two-day events may have the disadvantage that participants may experience difficulties in retaining all the relevant information about disputation and other important techniques. Marathon sessions can be quite exhausting for the participants and the counsellors alike. As institutions and private health insurance companies are now keen on cost-effectiveness the closed group run over six to twelve sessions is likely to become the option of choice. It has many advantages; for example, with the same group members there is less need to repeat explanations of the ABCDE paradigm or demonstrations of techniques such as relaxation or biofeedback methods. The optimum number of clients in such a group is normally between six and twelve. When taking a purely educational approach, many more members can be accommodated.

Although REBT stress counselling groups may focus on specific disorders such as anxiety, phobias or other stress-related complaints, one of the main criteria for screen-ing out potential group members is whether the client can participate in an appropriate manner. Compulsive talkers who may dominate the group session are excluded unless they are willing to change their behaviour. Individuals may be highly disturbed but if they are able to contribute to the group without being disruptive then they are not automatically excluded. Therefore many individuals who have been labelled as psychotic may be able to attend if they fulfil the main criteria of contribut-ing to the group's task and acting appropriately. If an individual becomes highly disruptive once on a programme then the counsellor would generally need to refer the person to individual counselling and exclude the person from the group.[32]

Whatever format is chosen, REBT stress counselling groups tend to be run on similar lines. At the first meeting, an explanation is given of the role of the counsellor, i.e. group leader who will be taking an active-directive approach, will be helping participants to change their self-disturbing Irrational Beliefs, and will teach a variety of stress management techniques such as relaxation and imagery exercises. Unlike other forms of therapy, the REBT group stress counsellor is not a facilitator. The counsellor negotiates suitable ground rules such as time-keeping, and confidentiality of personal information. The confidentiality rule does not extend to the sharing of stress management techniques members have learnt with their family and friends. In fact, rational proselytizing is actively encouraged as clients who teach others rational thinking and behaviour tend to become more convinced of the underlying philosophy.[33]

During the first session the counsellor gives a presentation on the ABCDEs of REBT. It is helpful to demonstrate to the group how holding musturbatory beliefs can elevate stress levels in a specific situation in contrast to holding preferential beliefs. If this is not undertaken at an early stage of therapy members may not see the point of disputing Irrational Beliefs. Either a problem from a group member could be used or an example of an ABC chain that most people can relate to is chosen instead such as the emotional consequences of arriving somewhere late. This can be illustrated diagrammatically on a whiteboard or a flip chart or on a handout as below:

A...Arriving late for an important meeting
B...I must not arrive late but if I do
    it would be awful and
    I could not stand it
C...

A typical dialogue the stress counsellor uses to describe the situation is below.

Counsellor:	I would like you all to imagine arriving late for an important meeting. (Counsellor points to the flip chart.) Is anybody having any difficulty?
John:	That's easy. It only happened last week to me!
Sue:	It only happened today to me. I thought I was going to turn up here late (laughs).
Counsellor:	OK. We call this situation the activating event or 'A' for short. OK. Now imagine you hold the following beliefs about turning up late: 'I MUST not arrive late but if I do it would be awful and I could not stand it.' (Counsellor points to the beliefs on the flip chart.) How would you feel?
Jayne:	I do hold those beliefs! I would feel really anxious. (The counsellor writes 'anxiety' alongside the 'C' on the flip chart.)
Counsellor:	What does everybody else think they would feel? (The counsellor is ensuring that everybody understands the model and can imagine the situation.)
Paul:	I'd feel nothing. I don't care if I turn up late anywhere.
Counsellor:	That's an interesting point, Paul. I'll come back to that later. However, just

for the purpose of this exercise can you really have a go at imagining that you do hold these beliefs which we call 'B'. (Counsellor then goes around the group to ensure that the other members can relate to this exercise.) If I held on to these beliefs and I arrived late I would probably appear very nervous and act in a clumsy manner. Can anybody relate to this additional behavioural consequence or 'C' as we call it?

Mitch: I remember being late for an important presentation I had to give. I was so nervous that I dropped all of the acetates on to the floor. I felt so stupid.

Counsellor: That was a good example, Mitch, of how becoming anxious in a situation tends to reduce performance. You also raised an interesting point about thinking you were stupid. However, if I may, I'll come back to that later.

Now, can you all imagine the same situation but this time you are telling yourself something different. (Counsellor turns over to another pre-prepared ABC sheet.)

This time you are telling yourself: 'It's strongly preferable to arrive on time but if I don't, it's bad but not awful, it's certainly not the end of my world and I can still stand it.' How do you feel this time?

Mitch: If I really could believe it, which I don't, I would feel less anxious.

Sue: I would probably just feel concerned. (The counsellor writes 'concern' next to the 'C' on the second sheet.)

Counsellor: Now can you see how it is not the 'A', in this case arriving late, that causes 'C', but what you think about 'A' that largely contributes to the 'C'?

At this stage the counsellor answers any queries the group has and then describes the relevance of the DE of the ABCDEs.

Plenty of time needs to be set aside for this activity. Then if there is still sufficient time left in the session, the counsellor can demonstrate the complete ABCDE process with an example from a group member. In the example above, the counsellor may decide to return to Mitch who gave an example of self-damnation and illustrate how even though he may have acted stupidly the behaviour does not mean that he is stupid. The counsellor may also discuss why Paul felt 'nothing'.

In the first session it is usually a good idea to avoid using an example from the group which involves procrastination as the underlying anxiety may not always be easy to demonstrate. However, this depends largely upon the experience and skill of the counsellor. As the first session can set a precedent, it is important for you to encourage the group members to participate and not just expect the counsellor to do the majority of the talking. At the end of the first session a useful homework assignment exercise to set the entire group is appropriate bibliotherapy. Books or short booklets, such as those by Dryden and Gordon, are recommended at this stage as this helps to orientate the members into REBT stress counselling.[34]

If the group meets weekly, the counsellor will usually negotiate a relevant homework assignment with each client. The counsellor will check up on how the client got on with the assignment at the next meeting. The counsellor may spend some time explaining to the group the importance of undertaking homework assignments if they really want to manage stress. Usually some of the group do not undertake their homework assignments as they cannot see their relevance to changing themselves. A typical explanation and discussion of this issue is below.

Counsellor:	In REBT we believe that the other 166 hours outside of the therapeutic two hours in every week are just as important. This is one of the main reasons why we always recommend that clients undertake homework assignments in between sessions. I would like to give you an analogy. How many of you drive a car (or automobile)?
Paul:	I've been driving for years.
Mitch:	I passed only recently.
Sue:	I've now failed twice.
Counsellor:	OK. So you all have some idea about driving cars. Think back to your first driving lesson. For most people it wasn't easy.
Sue:	You're not joking! I must have stalled it at least five times.
Counsellor:	Good. I'm glad you can recall it so well, Sue. Now just imagine that your favourite uncle, aunt or friend taught you how to drive. After many driving lessons you finally take your driving test and unfortunately fail it. Then you decide to have professional driving lessons and the instructor tells you that you are driving incorrectly, for example, not checking the mirror in the correct manner at the right time. Now imagine the difficulty you would experience having to relearn how to drive correctly.
Sue:	This actually happened to me. It's been impossible!
Counsellor:	(laughs): This is quite a common problem. Now let's relate this to homework assignments. Just imagine how many hours and years of your lives you have been thinking the way you all do in this room. Twenty years, 30 years, 40 years, and 50 years for some of you. Up to 50 years thinking in ways that exacerbate stress. Think of all the daily practice you've all had thinking in a way that causes you all so much distress. Do you honestly believe that just attending a stress counselling group once a week for two hours is going to make much impact on your crazy thinking deficits?
Paul:	Put that way, no. I just hadn't thought of it like that before. I've actually spent 45 years practising how to escalate my stress levels.
Counsellor:	Can you see why we believe that the other 166 hours of a week when you are not here are so important?
Mitch:	I can now.
Counsellor:	Incidentally Mitch, can you imagine what would have happened if you turned up on the day of your driving test having had NO lessons at all? What would have happened?
Mitch:	I definitely would have failed.
Counsellor:	Absolutely right! And this also applies to REBT. If you don't regularly practise your new thinking, feeling and behaving skills you are more likely to experience stress when the next difficulty arises. In the same way with practice you will automatically slam your brakes on if somebody walks out in front of you, eventually these new REBT skills start to occur more instinctively. But it takes hard work and practice.

Each week the counsellor deals with the problems and stress scenarios raised by the individual group members. After a few sessions, once the group members have grasped the ABCDEs of REBT, the counsellor encourages them to dispute each other's Irrational Beliefs in the session. The counsellor acts as a guide to keep the group on track and avoid any unnecessary departures from the basic ABCDEs of REBT.

Sessions often start with the counsellor asking the following opening question:

Counsellor: Who would like to discuss a problem today?
Paul: I do. I've got a presentation to do at work next week in front of the Board of Directors. I'm really feeling stressed about it.
Jayne: I've got one too. I have to fly to New York on work in a fortnight. You know how I hate flying. I just couldn't stand having another panic attack.
Counsellor: Anybody else? No. OK we'll start with Paul's problem.

In addition, the counsellor may set small group activities that focus on skills practice or, when necessary, she/he teaches imagery and relaxation techniques and time management and assertiveness skills. The counsellor discourages members from probing activating events too deeply as this leaves less time for disputation of the individual's Irrational Beliefs and the setting of appropriate homework assignments.

Occasionally a member stays silent or does not bring problems to therapy. Assuming that the client is not highly disturbed, the counsellor will usually bring the person into the conversation using a variety of methods, for example, 'Jayne, can you relate to Mitch's problem?' or 'Jayne, have you ever experienced a similar problem?' or 'You've been rather quiet today. What's going through your mind at this very instant?' If the client is avoiding discussing her own problems or talking in the group, then this can be investigated in ABCDE terms.[35]

If the stress therapy groups are open ended and not limited to a fixed number of sessions then, as old members leave, the counsellor needs to explain the ABCDEs of REBT to all new members on joining. However, we have found that experienced members can usually be encouraged to explain the rationale of REBT to the new members. Once again, this rational proselytizing appears to help reinforce the group members' own beliefs in the REBT approach and helps to orientate the new members.

NOTES

1. DiMattia, 1991, 1993; Ellis, 1972b, 1974b, 1994a; Ellis and Blum, 1967; Ellis and DiMattia, 1991a, 1991b; Neenan, 1993a, 1993b; Palmer, 1993a, 1995; Wessler and Wessler, 1980.
2. Sigman, 1992.
3. Adapted from Cooper, Cooper and Eaker, 1988.
4. Allison, Cooper and Reynolds, 1989.
5. Adapted from Palmer, 1993a.
6. Sloan and Cooper, 1986.
7. Quick and Quick, 1984.
8. Friedman and Ulmer, 1985.
9. Cowen, 1982.
10. Cox, Gotts, Boot and Kerr, 1988.
11. Cox, Leather and Cox, 1990.
12. Palmer, 1995, p. 46.

13. Cooper and Cartwright, 1994.
14. Evans and Reynolds, 1993; Palmer, 1993a.
15. Allison, Cooper and Reynolds, 1989.
16. Cooper, Sloan and Williams, 1988; Palmer, 1995.
17. Palmer and Dryden, 1995.
18. Baldon and Ellis, 1993; Clarke and Palmer, 1994; DiMattia and Mennen, 1990; Dryden and Gordon, 1990a, 1992, 1993a; Palmer and Dryden, 1996; Palmer and Strickland, 1995.
19. Palmer, 1995, pp. 48–9.
20. Palmer and Dryden, 1995.
21. Cooper, Cooper and Eaker, 1988.
22. Ellis, 1991a.
23. Palmer and Dryden, 1995.
24. Kushnir and Malkinson, 1993, p. 199.
25. Ellis and DiMattia, 1991a, p. 1.
26. Ellis and DiMattia, 1991a, pp. 4–6.
27. Wessler and Wessler, 1980.
28. Lazarus, 1981, p. 203.
29. Forsyth, 1991; Yalom, 1985.
30. Ellis, 1974b.
31. Ellis, 1974b, p. 20.
32. Wessler and Wessler, 1980.
33. Bard, 1973; Palmer and Dryden, 1995.
34. Dryden and Gordon, 1990a, 1992.
35. Wessler and Wessler, 1980.

AFTERWORD
Training in Rational Emotive Behaviour Therapy

We believe it is important for the professional development of both trainee and experienced counsellors and therapists to undertake further training to broaden their experience and to keep up to date in the rapidly expanding field of counselling. Training workshops are run by qualified and experienced REBT practitioners and cover a wide range of applications of REBT in counselling, clinical and industrial settings.

The Albert Ellis Institute for Rational Emotive Behavior Therapy (formerly the Institute for Rational-Emotive Therapy) in New York offers a comprehensive range of services including adult education workshops and multi-session courses, professional training programmes, consulting services for universities, corporations and other organizations, and a bookstore stocking publications and audiovisual materials for professional and educational use. For information, contact:

> The Albert Ellis Institute for Rational Emotive Behavior Therapy
> 45 East 65th Street
> New York
> NY 10021-6593
> USA
> Tel: (001) 212 535 0822
> e-mail: info@rebt.org

If you would like details of training courses in REBT held in England contact:

1. Centre for Rational Emotive Behaviour Therapy
   156 Westcombe Hill
   Blackheath
   London SE3 7DH
   Tel: 0181293 4114
   Fax: 0181293 1441

2. Professor Windy Dryden
   Department of Psychology
   Goldsmiths College
   New Cross
   London SE14 6NW
   Tel: 0171919 7872

The Albert Ellis Institute, the principal centre for REBT training, can also provide details of Affiliated Training Centres elsewhere in the United States and in other countries. If you would like further information please contact:

CANADA

1. Centre for Rational-Emotive Therapy
   Kurt Fuerst, PhD
   912-170 Laurier Avenue
   West Ottawa
   Ontario K1P SV5
   Canada
   Tel: (001) 613 231-6556
2. Sam Klarreich, PhD
   172 King Street East
   Toronto
   Ontario M5A 1J3
   Canada
   Tel: (001) 416 861-9322

AUSTRALIA

   Australian Institute for RET
   118 Balcombe Road
   Mentone
   Victoria 3804
   Australia
   Tel: (0061) 9585-1881

GERMANY

   Deutsches Institut für RET und Kognitive Verhaltenstherapie (DIREKT)
   Muellersweg 14
   D-97249 Eisengen
   Germany
   Tel: (0049) 931-8 15 56

ISRAEL

Israeli Centre for RET
27 Gluskin Street
PO Box 1006
Rehovot 76470
Israel
Tel: (00972) 8 463165

ITALY

Institute for RET-Italy
Via G. Trezza, 12
37129 Verona
Italy
Tel: (0039) 45-596993

FRANCE

Institut Francais de Thérapie Cognitive
55 Passage du Grade Turc
1400 Caen
France
Tel: (0033) 2-31-500149

MEXICO

Instituto de Terapia Racional-Emotiva de México
Rincón del Bosque #25
Colonia Polanco, Mexico DF
Mexico
Tel: (0052) 5-255-3611

NETHERLANDS

Institut voor Rationeel-Emotieve Training
Postbus 316
2000 AH Haarlem
Netherlands
Tel: (0031) 23-5328817

Finally, the authors would be interested to hear your views and experience of the REBT approach to Stress Counselling and Stress Management. Please write to:
    Albert Ellis at The Albert Ellis Institute, New York
    or to:
    Jack Gordon, Michael Neenan and Stephen Palmer at the Centre for Rational Emotive Behaviour Therapy, London
    (addresses fully listed above).

References

(Items marked with a * are mainly self-help materials on REBT.)

Abrams, M. and Ellis, A. (1994) Rational emotive behaviour therapy in the treatment of stress. *British Journal of Guidance and Counselling*, **22** (1), 39–50.

Allison, T., Cooper, C.L. and Reynolds, P. (1989) Stress counselling in the workplace. *The Psychologist*, 384–8.

American Psychiatric Association (1994) *Diagnostic and Statistical Manual of Mental Disorders* (4th edn). Washington, DC: Author.

*Baldon, A. and Ellis, A. (1993) *RET Problem Solving Workbook*. New York: Institute for Rational-Emotive Therapy.

Bard, J.A. (1973) Rational proselytising. *Rational Living*, **12** (1), 2–6.

Barlow, D.H. (1988) *Anxiety and its Disorders*. New York: Guilford.

Beck, A.T. (1976) *Cognitive Therapy and the Emotional Disorders*. New York: International Universities Press.

Beck, A.T. and Emery, G. (1985) *Anxiety Disorders and Phobias: A Cognitive Perspective*. New York: Basic Books.

Beck, A.T., Freeman, A. and Associates (1990) *Cognitive Therapy of Personality Disorders*. New York: Guilford.

Beck, A.T., Rush, A., Shaw, B. and Emery, G. (1979) *Cognitive Therapy of Depression*. New York: Guilford.

Beck, A.T., Steer, R.A., Kovacs, M. and Garrison, B. (1985) Hopelessness and eventual suicide: A ten year prospective study of patients hospitalized with suicidal ideation. *American Journal of Psychiatry*, **42** (5), 559–63.

Benson, H. (1975) *The Relaxation Response*. New York: Morrow.

Bressler, J. (1988) Eating disorders and obesity. *Journal of Rational-Emotive and Cognitive-Behavior Therapy*, **6** (1 & 2), 9–22.

Burish, T.G. (1981) EMG biofeedback in the treatment of stress-related disorders. In C. Prokop and L.A. Bradley (eds), *Medical Psychology: Contributions to Behavioral Science* (pp. 395–421).

Clark, D.M. (1989) Anxiety states. In K. Hawton, P.M. Salkovskis, J. Kirk and D.M. Clark (eds), *Cognitive Behaviour Therapy for Psychiatric Problems* (pp. 52–6). Oxford: Oxford University Press.

*Clark, D. and Palmer, S. (1994) *How to Manage Stress*. Cambridge: National Extension College.

Cooper, C.L. and Cartwright, S. (1994) Stress-management interventions in the workplace: Stress counselling and stress audits. *British Journal of Guidance and Counselling*, **22** (1), 65–73.

Cooper, C.L., Cooper, R. and Eaker, L. (1988) *Living with Stress*. Harmondsworth: Penguin Books.

Cooper, C.L., Sloan, S. and Williams, S. (1988) *Occupational Stress Indicator: Management Guide*. Windsor: NFER-Nelson.

Cowen, E.L. (1982) Help is where you find it. *American Psychologist*, **37**, 385–95.

Cox, T., Gotts, G., Boot, N. and Kerr, J. (1988) Physical exercise, employee fitness and the management of health at work. *Work and Stress*, **2** (1), 71–6.

Cox, T., Leather, P. and Cox, S. (1990) Stress, health and organisations. *Occupational Health Review*, **23**, 13–18.

Crawford, T. and Ellis, A. (1989) A dictionary of rational-emotive feelings and behaviors. *Journal of Rational-Emotive and Cognitive Behavior Therapy*, **7** (1), 3–27.

DiGiuseppe, R. (1991) A rational-emotive model of assessment. In M.E. Bernard (ed.), *Using Rational-Emotive Therapy Successfully: A Practitioner's Guide* (pp. 151–72). New York and London: Plenum.

DiMattia, D. (1991) RET in the workplace. In M.E. Bernard (ed.), *Using Rational-Emotive Therapy Effectively: A Practitioner's Guide*. New York and London: Plenum.

DiMattia, D. (1993) RET in the workplace. *Journal of Rational-Emotive and Cognitive-Behavior Therapy*, **11** (2), 61–3.

DiMattia, D.J. and Mennen, S. (1990) *Rational Effectiveness Training: Increasing Personal Productivity at Work*. New York: Institute for Rational-Emotive Therapy.

Dolan, C.A., Sherwood, A. and Light, K.C. (1992) Cognitive coping strategies and blood pressure responses to real-life stress in healthy young men. *Health Psychology*, **11** (4), 233–40.

Dryden, W. (1987) *Counselling Individuals: The Rational-Emotive Approach*. London: Taylor and Francis.

Dryden, W. (1989) The use of chaining in rational-emotive therapy. *Journal of Rational-Emotive and Cognitive-Behavior Therapy*, **7** (2), 59–66.

Dryden, W. (1990a) *Creativity in Rational-Emotive Therapy*. Loughton, Essex: Gale Centre Publications.

Dryden, W. (1990b) *Rational-Emotive Counselling in Action*. London: Sage.

Dryden, W. (1990c) *Dealing with Anger Problems: Rational-Emotive Therapeutic Interventions*. Sarasota, FL: Professional Resource Exchange, Inc.

Dryden, W. (1991) *A Dialogue with Albert Ellis: Against Dogma*. Milton Keynes: Open University Press.

Dryden, W. (1994a) *Progress in Rational Emotive Behaviour Therapy*. London: Whurr.

*Dryden, W. (1994b) *Overcoming Guilt*. London: Sheldon.

Dryden, W. (1995a) *Preparing for Client Change in Rational Emotive Behaviour Therapy*. London: Whurr.

Dryden, W. (1995b) *Brief Rational Emotive Behaviour Therapy*. London: Wiley.

*Dryden, W. (1996) *Overcoming Anger*. London: Sheldon.

Dryden, W. and DiGiuseppe, R. (1990) *A Primer on Rational-Emotive Therapy*. Champaign, IL: Research Press.

*Dryden, W. and Gordon, J. (1990a) *Think Your Way to Happiness*. London: Sheldon.

Dryden, W. and Gordon, J. (1990b) *What Is Rational-Emotive Therapy? A Personal and Practical Guide*. Loughton, Essex, England: Gale Publications.

*Dryden, W. and Gordon, J. (1992) *Think Rationally: A Brief Guide to Overcoming Your Emotional Problems*. London: Centre for Rational Emotive Behaviour Therapy.

*Dryden, W. and Gordon, J. (1993a) *Peak Performance: Become More Effective at Work*. Didcot: Mercury Business Books.

*Dryden, W. and Gordon, J. (1993b) *Beating the Comfort Trap*. London: Sheldon.

Dryden, W. and Neenan, M. (1995) *Dictionary of Rational Emotive Behaviour Therapy*. London: Whurr.

Ellis, A. (1962) *Reason and Emotion in Psychotherapy*. Secaucus, NJ: Citadel.

Ellis, A. (1965) *The Treatment of Borderline and Psychotic Individuals*. New York: Institute for Rational-Emotive Therapy. (Rev. edn 1988.)

*Ellis, A. (1972a) *Psychotherapy and the Value of a Human Being*. New York: Institute for Rational-Emotive Therapy. (Reprinted in A. Ellis and W. Dryden, *The Essential Albert Ellis*. New York: Springer, 1990.)

Ellis, A. (1972b) *Executive Leadership: A Rational-Emotive Approach*. New York: Institute for Rational-Emotive Therapy.

Ellis, A. (1972c) Helping people get better: rather than feel better. *Rational Living*, 7 (2), 2–9.

Ellis, A. (1973) *Humanistic Psychotherapy: The Rational-Emotive Approach*. New York: McGraw-Hill.

*Ellis, A. (1974a) *Disputing Irrational Beliefs (DIBS)*. New York: Institute for Rational-Emotive Therapy.

Ellis, A. (1974b) Rational-Emotive Therapy in groups. *Rational Living*, 9 (1), 15–22.

Ellis, A. (1976) The biological basis of human irrationality. *Journal of Individual Psychology*, 32, 145–68. (Reprinted, Institute for Rational-Emotive Therapy, New York, 1976.)

Ellis, A. (1977a) The basic clinical theory of rational-emotive therapy. In A. Ellis and R. Greiger (eds), *Handbook of Rational-Emotive Therapy*, Vol. 1. New York: Springer.

Ellis, A. (1977b) Characteristics of psychotic and borderline individuals. In A. Ellis and R. Greiger (eds), *Handbook of Rational-Emotive Therapy*, Vol. 1 (pp. 177–86). New York: Springer.

Ellis, A. (1977c) Intimacy in psychotherapy. *Rational Living*, 12 (2), 13–19.

*Ellis, A., (1977d) *Fun as Psychotherapy*. (Cassette recording.) New York: Institute for Rational-Emotive Therapy.

*Ellis, A. (1977e) *A Garland of Rational Humorous Songs*. (Cassette recording and songbook.) New York: Institute for Rational-Emotive Therapy.

Ellis, A. (1977f) Skill training in counselling and psychotherapy. *Canadian Counsellor*, 12 (1), 30–5.

Ellis, A. (1978) What people can do for themselves to cope with stress. In C.L. Cooper and R. Payne, *Stress at Work* (pp. 209–22). Chichester and New York: John Wiley.

Ellis, A. (1979a) Rational-Emotive Therapy: Research data that supports the clinical and personality hypotheses of RET and other modes of cognitive-behavior therapy. In A. Ellis and J.M. Whiteley (eds), *Theoretical and Empirical Foundations of Rational-Emotive Therapy* (pp. 101–73). Monterey, CA: Brooks/Cole.

Ellis, A. (1979b) The issue of force and energy in behavioral change. *Journal of Contemporary Psychotherapy*, 10 (2), 83–97. (Reprinted in W. Dryden (ed.), *Rational Emotive Behaviour Therapy: A Reader*. London: Sage, 1995).

*Ellis, A. (1979c) *The Intelligent Woman's Guide to Dating and Mating*. Secaucus, NJ: Lyle Stuart.

Ellis, A. (1979d) Discomfort anxiety: A new cognitive-behavioral construct. Part 1. *Rational Living*, 14 (2), 3–8.

Ellis, A. (1980) Discomfort anxiety: A new cognitive-behavioral construct. Part 2. *Rational Living*, 15 (1), 25–30.

Ellis, A. (1982) Intimacy in rational-emotive therapy. In M. Fisher and G. Striker (eds), *Intimacy*. New York: Plenum.

Ellis, A. (1983a) Failures in rational-emotive therapy. In E. Foa and P.M. Emmelkamp (eds), *Failures in Behavior Therapy* (pp. 159–71). New York: Wiley.

Ellis, A. (1983b) The philosophic implications and dangers of some popular behavior therapy techniques. In M. Rosenbaum, C.M. Franks and Y. Jaffe (eds), *Perspectives in Behavior Therapy in the Eighties* (pp. 138–51). New York: Plenum.

*Ellis, A. (1983c) *The Case Against Religiosity*. New York: Institute for Rational-Emotive Therapy.

Ellis, A. (1985a) *Overcoming Resistance: Rational-Emotive Therapy with Difficult Clients*. New York: Springer.

Ellis, A. (1985b) Love and its problems. In A. Ellis and M.E. Bernard (eds), *Clinical Applications of Rational-Emotive Therapy* (pp. 31–53). New York: Plenum.

Ellis, A. (1985c) Intellectual fascism. *Journal of Rational-Emotive Therapy*, 3 (1), 3–12.

Ellis, A. (1986) Anxiety about anxiety: The use of hypnosis with rational-emotive therapy. In E.T. Dowd and J.M. Healy (eds), *Case Studies in Hypnotherapy* (pp. 3–11). New York: Guilford. (Reprinted in A. Ellis and W. Dryden, *The Practice of Rational-Emotive Therapy*. New York: Springer, 1987.)

Ellis, A. (1987a) The use of rational humorous songs in psychotherapy. In W.F. Fry, Jr and W.A. Salameh (eds), *Handbook of Humor and Psychotherapy* (pp. 265–87). Sarasota, FL: Professional Resource Exchange.

Ellis, A. (Speaker) (1987b) *The Enemies of Humanism – What Makes Them Tick?* (Cassette recording, no. 108.) New York and Alexandria, VA: Audio Transcripts.

Ellis, A. (1987c) Testament of a humanist. *Free Inquiry*, 7 (2), 21.

Ellis, A. (1987d) Ask Dr Ellis. *Journal of Rational-Emotive Therapy*, 5 (2), 135–7.

*Ellis, A. (1988) *How to Stubbornly Refuse to Make Yourself Miserable about Anything – Yes, Anything!* Secaucus, NJ: Lyle Stuart.

Ellis, A. (1989) *The Treatment of Psychotic and Borderline Individuals with RET*. New York: Institute for Rational-Emotive Therapy. (Original work published 1965.)

Ellis, A. (1990a) Special features of rational-emotive therapy. In W. Dryden and R. DiGiuseppe, *A Primer on Rational-Emotive Therapy* (pp. 79–93). Champaign, IL: Research Press.

Ellis, A. (1990b) A rational-emotive approach to peace. Paper delivered at the 98th Annual Convention of the American Psychological Society, Boston.

Ellis, A. (1990c) Is rational-emotive therapy (RET) 'rationalist' or 'constructivist'? *Journal of Rational-Emotive and Cognitive-Behavior Therapy*, 8 (3), 169–93.

Ellis, A. (1991a) *Using RET Effectively: Reflections and Interview*. In M.E. Bernard (ed.), *Using Rational-Emotive Therapy Effectively* (pp. 1–33). New York: Plenum.

Ellis, A. (1991b) The revised ABCs of rational-emotive therapy. In J. Zeig (ed.), *Evolution of Psychotherapy: II*. New York: Brunner/Mazel. (Expanded version in *Journal of Rational-Emotive and Cognitive Behavior Therapy*, 1991, 9 (3), 139–72.)

Ellis, A. (1991c) Achieving self-actualization. In A. Jones and R. Crandall (eds), *Handbook of Self-actualization*. Corte Madera, CA: Select Press.

Ellis, A. (1992a) Brief therapy: The rational-emotive method. In S.H. Budman, M.F. Hoyt and S. Friedman (eds), *The First Session in Brief Therapy*. New York: Guilford.

Ellis, A. (1992b) Group rational-emotive and cognitive-behavior therapy. *International Journal of Group Therapy*, 42, 63–80.

Ellis, A. (1993a) Rational-emotive imagery: RET version. In M.E. Bernard and J. Wolfe (eds), *The RET Resource Book for Practitioners* (pp. 11–18). New York: Institute for Rational-Emotive Therapy.

Ellis, A. (1993b) Vigorous RET disputing. In M.E. Bernard and J. Wolfe (eds), *The RET Resource Book for Practitioners* (pp. 11–17). New York: Institute for Rational-Emotive Therapy.

Ellis, A. (Speaker) (1993c) *Overcoming Stress and Anxiety*. London: Centre for Rational Emotive Behaviour Therapy.

Ellis, A. (1993d) Rational-emotive imagery and hypnosis. In J.W. Rhue, S.J. Lynn and I. Kirsch (eds), *Handbook of Clinical Hypnosis* (pp. 173–86). Washington, DC: American Psychological Association.

Ellis, A. (1994a) *Reason and Emotion in Psychotherapy* (Revised and updated). New York: Carol Publishing.

Ellis, A. (1994b) Post-traumatic stress disorder (PTSD): A rational emotive behavioral theory. *Journal of Rational-Emotive and Cognitive-Behavior Therapy*, 12 (1), 3–25.

Ellis, A. (1994c) Rational emotive behavior therapy approaches to obsessive-compulsive disorder (OCD). *Journal of Rational-Emotive and Cognitive-Behavior Therapy*, 12 (2), 121–41.

Ellis, A. (1994d) The treatment of borderline personalities with rational emotive behavior therapy. *Journal of Rational-Emotive and Cognitive-Behavior Therapy*, 12 (2), 101–19.

Ellis, A. (1995a) Fundamentals of Rational Emotive Behaviour Therapy for the 1990s. In W. Dryden (ed.), *Rational Emotive Behaviour Therapy: A Reader* (pp. 1–30). London: Sage Publications.

Ellis, A. (1995b) Albert Ellis on rational emotive behavior therapy and counselling psychology. In S. Palmer, W. Dryden, A. Ellis and R. Yapp (eds), *Rational Interviews*. London: Centre for Rational Emotive Behaviour Therapy.

Ellis, A. (1995c) Rational-emotive approaches to overcoming resistance. In W. Dryden (ed.), *Rational Emotive Behaviour Therapy: A Reader* (pp. 184–211). London: Sage. (Originally published in A. Ellis and R. Greiger with contributors, *Handbook of Rational-Emotive Therapy*, Vol. 2 (pp. 221–45). Springer, New York, 1986.)

Ellis, A. (1996) *Better, Deeper and More Enduring Brief Therapy*. New York: Brunner/Mazel.

Ellis, A. and Abrahms, E. (1978) *Brief Psychotherapy in Medical and Health Practice*. New York: Springer.

*Ellis, A. and Abrams, M. (1994) *How to Cope with a Fatal Illness*. New York: Barricade Books.

*Ellis, A. and Becker, I. (1982) *A Guide to Personal Happiness*. North Hollywood, CA: Wilshire.

Ellis, A. and Blum, M.L. (1967) Rational Training: A new method of facilitating management labor relations. *Psychological Reports*, 20, 1267–84.

Ellis, A. and DiMattia, D. (1991a) *Rational Effectiveness Training: A New Method of Facilitating Management and Labor Relations*. New York: Institute for Rational-Emotive Therapy.

*Ellis, A. and DiMattia, D. (1991b) *Self Management: Strategies for Personal Success*. New York: Institute for Rational-Emotive Therapy.

Ellis, A. and Dryden, W. (1987) *The Practice of Rational Emotive Behavior Therapy* (2nd edn). New York: Springer.

Ellis, A. and Dryden, W. (1990) *The Essential Albert Ellis*. New York: Springer.

Ellis, A. and Dryden, W. (1991) *A Dialogue with Albert Ellis: Against Dogma*. Stony Stratford, Milton Keynes: Open University Press.

*Ellis, A. and Harper, R.A. (1975) *A New Guide to Rational Living*. North Hollywood, CA: Wilshire.

*Ellis, A. and Harper, R.A. (1997) *A Guide to Rational Living* (Revised and updated edn). North Hollywood, CA: Wilshire.

*Ellis, A. and Knaus, W.J. (1977) *Overcoming Procrastination*. New York: Institute for Rational-Emotive Therapy.

Ellis, A., McInerney, J.F., DiGiuseppe, R. and Yeager, R.J. (1988) *Rational-Emotive Therapy with Alcoholics and Substance Abusers*. New York: Pergamon.

*Ellis, A. and Velten, E. (1992) *When AA Doesn't Work for You: Rational Steps to Quitting Alcohol*. New York: Barricade Books.

Ellis, A. and Whiteley, J.M. (1979) *Theoretical and Empirical Foundations of Rational-Emotive Therapy*. Monterey, CA: Brooks/Cole.

Ellis, A. and Yeager, R. (1989) *Why Some Therapies Don't Work: The Dangers of Transpersonal Psychology*. Buffalo, NY: Prometheus Books.

Esterling, B.A., Kiecolt-Glaser, J.K., Bodnar, J.C. and Glaser, R. (1994) Chronic stress, social support, and persistent alterations in the natural killer cell response to cytokines in older adults. *Health Psychology*, **13** (4), 291–8.

Evans, B. and Reynolds, P. (1993) Stress counselling: A client-centred approach. *Stress News*, **5** (1), 2–6.

Fairburn, C. (1995) (Interview) Living in fear of being fat. *The Times*, 25 April.

Fairburn, C.G. and Cooper, P.J. (1989) Eating disorders. In K. Hawton, P.M. Salkovskis, J. Kirk and D.M. Clark (eds), *Cognitive Behaviour Therapy for Psychiatric Problems* (pp. 277–314). Oxford: Oxford University Press.

Fennell, M.J.V. (1989) Depression. In K. Hawton, P.M. Salkovskis, J. Kirk and D.M. Clark (eds), *Cognitive Behaviour Therapy for Psychiatric Problems* (pp. 169–234). Oxford: Oxford University Press.

Forsyth, D.R. (1991) Changes in therapeutic groups. In C.R. Snyder and D.R. Forsyth (eds), *Handbook of Social and Clinical Psychology* (pp. 664–80). New York: Pergamon.

Frank, J.D. (1973) *Persuasion and Healing* (rev. edn). Baltimore: The Johns Hopkins University Press.

Friedman, M. and Ulmer, D. (1985) *Treating Type A Behaviour and Your Heart*. London: Michael Joseph.

Greenwood, V. (1985) RET and substance abuse. In A. Ellis and M.E. Bernard (eds), *Clinical Applications of Rational-Emotive Therapy* (pp. 209–35). New York: Plenum.

Hauck, P. (1966) The neurotic agreement in psychotherapy. *Rational Living*, **1** (1), 31–4.

*Hauck, P. (1973) *Overcoming Depression*. Philadelphia: Westminster.

*Hauck, P. (1982) *How to Do What You Want to Do*. London: Sheldon.

*Hauck, P. (1991) *Overcoming the Rating Game*. London: Sheldon.

Hempel, C.G. (1966) *Philosophy of Natural Sciences*. Englewood Cliffs, NJ: Prentice-Hall.

Janoff-Bulman, R. (1985) The aftermath of victimization: Rebuilding shattered assumptions. In C.R. Figley (ed.), *Trauma and its Wake*. New York: Brunner/Mazel.

Klarreich, S.H. (1985) Stress: An interpersonal approach. In S.H. Klarreich, J.L. Francek and C.E. Moore (eds), *The Human Resources Handbook* (pp. 304–18). New York: Praeger.

Korzybski, A. (1933) *Science and Sanity*. San Francisco: International Society of General Semantics.

Kuhn, T. (1970) *The Structure of Scientific Revolutions* (2nd edn). Chicago: University of Chicago Press.

Kushnir, T. and Malkinson, R. (1993) A rational-emotive group intervention for preventing and coping with stress among safety officers. *Journal of Rational-Emotive and Cognitive-Behavior Therapy*, **11** (4), 195–206.

Lakatos, I. (1970) Falsification and the methodology of scientific programmes. In I. Lakatos and A. Musgrave (eds), *Criticism and the Growth of Knowledge* (pp. 91–196).

Lazarus, A.A. (1977) Toward an egoless state of being. In A. Ellis and R. Grieger (eds), *Handbook of Rational-Emotive Therapy*. New York: McGraw-Hill.

Lazarus, A.A. (1981) *The Practice of Multimodal Therapy*. New York: McGraw-Hill.

Lazarus, A.A. and Mayne, T.J. (1990) Relaxation: Some limitations, side effects and proposed solutions. *Psychotherapy*, **27** (2), 261–6.

Leaf, R.C. and DiGiuseppe, R. (1992) Review of Beck et al., *Cognitive Therapy of Personality Disorders*. *Journal of Rational-Emotive and Cognitive-Behavior Therapy*, **10** (2), 105–8.

Macaskill, N.D. (1989) Educating clients about rational-emotive therapy. In W. Dryden and P. Trower (eds), *Cognitive Psychotherapy: Stasis and Change* (pp. 87–98). London: Cassell. (Reprinted in W. Dryden (ed.), *Rational Emotive Behaviour Therapy: A Reader* (pp. 42–52). London: Sage, 1995.)

McCrea, C. (1991) Eating disorders. In W. Dryden and R. Rentoul (eds), *Adult Clinical Problems: A Cognitive-Behavioural Approach* (pp. 114–37). London: Routledge.

McKinnon, W., Weisse, C.S., Reynolds, C.P., Bowles, C.A. and Baum, A. (1989) Chronic stress, leukocyte subpopulations, and humor response to latent viruses. *Health Psychology*, 8, 389–402.

McMullin, R.E. (1986) *Handbook of Cognitive Therapy Techniques*. New York: Norton.

Martin, R.D. (1984) A critical review of the concept of stress in psychomatic medicine. *Perspectives in Biology and Medicine*, 27 (3), 443–63.

*Maultsby, M.C., Jr and Ellis, A. (1974) *Techniques for Using Rational-Emotive Imagery*. New York: Institute for Rational-Emotive Therapy.

Moore, R.H. (1993) Traumatic incident reduction: A cognitive-emotive treatment of post-traumatic stress disorder. In W. Dryden and L.K. Hill (eds), *Innovations in Rational-Emotive Therapy* (pp. 116–59). London: Sage.

Muran, E.M. and DiGiuseppe, R. (1994) Rape. In F.M. Dattilio and A. Freeman (eds), *Cognitive-Behavioural Strategies in Crisis Intervention* (pp. 67–103). New York: Guilford.

Neenan, M. (1993a) Rational-emotive therapy at work. *Stress News*, 5 (1), 7–10.

Neenan, M. (1993b) Using rational-emotive therapy in the workplace. *The Rational-Emotive Therapist*, 1 (1), 23–6.

Palmer, S. (1989) Occupational stress. *The Safety and Health Practitioner*, 7 (8), 15–18.

Palmer, S. (1990) Stress mapping: A visual technique to aid counselling or training. *Employee Counselling Today*, 2 (2), 9–12.

Palmer, S. (1993a) Organisational stress: Symptoms, causes and reduction. *Newsletter of the Society of Public Health*, November, 2–8.

Palmer, S. (1993b) Occupational stress: Its causes and alleviation. In W. Dekker (ed.), *Chief Executive International*. London: Sterling Publications.

Palmer, S. (1993c) Stress management interventions. *The Specialist (International)*, 4 (6), 35–9.

Palmer, S. (1993d) *Multimodal Techniques: Relaxation and Hypnosis*. London: Centre for Stress Management.

Palmer, S. (1995) A comprehensive approach to industrial rational emotive behaviour stress management workshops. *The Rational Emotive Behaviour Therapist*, 3 (1), 45–55.

Palmer, S. (1996) The multimodal approach: theory, assessment, techniques and interventions. In S. Palmer and W. Dryden (eds), *Stress Management and Counselling: Theory, Practice, Research and Methodology* (pp. 45–58). London: Cassell.

Palmer, S. and Burton, T. (1996) *Dealing with People Problems at Work*. Maidenhead: McGraw-Hill.

Palmer, S. and Dryden, W. (1995) *Counselling for Stress Problems*. London: Sage.

Palmer, S. and Dryden, W. (eds) (1996) *Stress Management and Counselling: Theory, Practice, Research and Methodology*. London: Cassell.

Palmer, S. and Ellis, A. (1995a) Brief therapy: Stephen Palmer interviews Albert Ellis. *The Rational Emotive Behaviour Therapist*, 3 (2) 68–71.

Palmer, S. and Ellis, A. (1995b) Stress counselling and management: Stephen Palmer interviews Albert Ellis. *The Rational Emotive Behaviour Therapist*, 3 (2), 82–6.

*Palmer, S. and Strickland, L. (1995) *Stress Management: A Quick Guide*. Cambridge: Daniels Publishing.

Popper, K.R. (1962) *Objective Knowledge*. London: Oxford.

Quick, J.C. and Quick, J.D. (1984) *Organisational Stress and Preventive Management*. New York: McGraw-Hill.

Reinecke, M.A. (1994) Suicide and depression. In F.M. Dattilio and A. Freeman (eds), *Cognitive-Behavioral Strategies in Crisis Intervention* (pp. 57–103). New York: Guilford.

Salkovskis, P.M. and Clark, D.M. (1991) Cognitive therapy for panic attacks. *Journal of Cognitive Psychotherapy*, 5 (3), 215–26.

Sichel, V. and Ellis, A. (1984) *REBT Self-Help Form*. New York: Institute for Rational-Emotive Therapy.

Sigman, A. (1992) The state of corporate health care. *Personnel Management*, February, 24–31.

Sloan, S. and Cooper, C. (1986) *Pilots Under Stress*. London: Routledge and Kegan Paul.

Wagenaar, J. and La Forge, J. (1994) Stress counselling theory and practice: A cautionary review. *Journal of Counselling and Development*, 73, September/October..

Walen, S.R., DiGiuseppe, R. and Dryden, W. (1992) *A Practitioner's Guide to Rational-Emotive Therapy* (2nd edn). New York: Oxford University Press.

Walen, S.R., DiGiuseppe, R. and Wessler, R.L. (1980) *A Practitioner's Guide to Rational-Emotive Therapy*. New York: Oxford University Press.

Warren, R. and Zgourides, G.D. (1991) *Anxiety Disorders: A Rational-Emotive Perspective*. New York: Pergamon.

Wessler, R.A. and Wessler, R.L. (1980) *The Principles and Practice of Rational-Emotive Therapy*. San Francisco: Jossey-Bass.

Wolpe, J. and Lazarus, A.A. (1966) *Behavior Therapy Techniques*. New York: Pergamon.

Woods, P.J. and Greiger, R.M. (1993) Bulimia: A case study with mediating cognitions and notes on a cognitive-behavioral analysis of eating disorders. *Journal of Rational-Emotive and Cognitive-Behavior Therapy*, 11 (3), 159–72.

Woods, P.J. and Muller, G.E. (1988) The contemplation of suicide: Its relationship to irrational beliefs in a client sample and the implications for long range suicide prevention. *Journal of Rational-Emotive and Cognitive-Behavior Therapy*, 6 (4), 236–58.

Yalom, I. (1995) *The Theory and Practice of Group Psychotherapy* (3rd edn). New York: Basic Books.

Yankura, J. and Dryden, W. (1990) *Doing RET: Albert Ellis in Action*. New York: Springer.

Young, H.S. (1974) *A Rational Counseling Primer*. New York: Institute for Rational-Emotive Therapy.

Young, H.S. (1988) Teaching rational self-value concepts to tough customers. In W. Dryden and P. Trower (eds), *Developments in Rational-Emotive Therapy* (pp. 132–58). Milton Keynes: Open University Press.

Young, J.E. and Lindeman, M.D. (1992) An integrative schema-focused model for personality disorders. *Journal of Cognitive Psychotherapy*, 6 (1), 11–23.

APPENDIX 1

REBT SELF-HELP FORM

Institute for Rational-Emotive Therapy
45 East 65th Street, New York, NY 10021
(212) 535-0822

(A) ACTIVATING EVENTS, thoughts, or feelings that happened just before I felt emotionally
disturbed or acted self-defeatingly:_____

_____

(C) CONSEQUENCE or CONDITIONS —disturbed feeling or self-defeating behavior – that I
produced and would like to change: _____

_____

(B) BELIEFS—Irrational BELIEFS (IBs) leading to my CONSEQUENCE (emotional disturbance or self-defeating behavior). Circle all that apply to these ACTIVATING EVENTS (A).	(D) DISPUTES for each circled IRRATIONAL BELIEF. Examples: "Why MUST I do very well?" "Where is it written that I am a BAD PERSON?" "Where is the evidence that I MUST be approved or accepted?"	(E) EFFECTIVE RATIONAL BELIEFS (RBs) to replace my IRRATIONAL BELIEFS (IBs). Examples: "I'd PREFER to do very well but I don't HAVE TO." "I am a PERSON WHO acted badly, not a BAD PERSON." "There is no evidence that I HAVE TO be approved though I would LIKE to be."
1. I MUST do well or very well!	....	....
2. I am a BAD OR WORTHLESS PERSON when I act weakly or stupidly.	....	....
3. I MUST be approved or accepted by people I find important!	....	....
4. I NEED to be loved by someone who matters to me a lot!	....	....
5. I am a BAD, UNLOVABLE PERSON if I get rejected.	....	....
6. People must treat me fairly and give me what I NEED!	....	....
7. People MUST live up to my expectations or it is TERRIBLE!	....	....

8. People who act immorally are undeserving, ROTTEN PEOPLE!		
9. I CAN'T STAND really bad things or very difficult people!		
10. My life MUST have few major hassles or troubles.		
11. It's AWFUL or HORRIBLE when major things don't go my way!		
12. I CAN'T STAND IT when life is really unfair!		
13. I NEED a good deal of immediate gratification and HAVE TO feel miserable when I don't get it!		
<u>Additional irrational Beliefs</u>:		

(F) FEELINGS and BEHAVIORS I experienced after arriving at my EFFECTIVE RATIONAL BELIEFS: _____

_____

I WILL WORK HARD TO REPEAT MY EFFECTIVE RATIONAL BELIEFS FORCEFULLY TO MYSELF ON MANY OCCASIONS SO THAT I CAN MAKE MYSELF LESS DISTURBED NOW AND ACT LESS SELF-DEFEATINGLY IN THE FUTURE.

Joyce Sichel, PhD and Albert Ellis, PhD   100 forms $10.00
1000 forms $80.00

APPENDIX 2
Assignment Task Sheet

Name _____ Date _ /_ /_ Negotiated with _____

Agreed task:

The therapeutic purpose(s) of the task:

Obstacles to carrying out the task – what obstacles, if any, stand in your way of completing this task and how you can overcome them:

1

2

3

Penalty:

Reward:

Signed: _____

APPENDIX 3

Techniques for Disputing Irrational Beliefs (DIBS)

Albert Ellis

If you want to increase your rationality and reduce your self-defeating irrational beliefs, you can spend at least ten minutes every day asking yourself the following questions and carefully thinking through (not merely parroting!) the healthy answers. Write down each question and your answers to it on a piece of paper; or else record the questions and your answers on a tape recorder.

1. WHAT SELF-DEFEATING IRRATIONAL BELIEF DO I WANT TO DISPUTE AND SURRENDER?
ILLUSTRATIVE ANSWER: I must receive love from someone for whom I really care.
2. CAN I RATIONALLY SUPPORT THIS BELIEF?
ILLUSTRATIVE ANSWER: No.
3. WHAT EVIDENCE EXISTS OF THE FALSENESS OF THIS BELIEF?
ILLUSTRATIVE ANSWER:
Many indications exist that the belief that I must receive love from someone for whom I really care is false:
a) No law of the universe exists that says that someone I care for *must* love me (although I would find it nice if that person did!).
b) If I do not receive love from one person, I can still get it from others and find happiness that way.
c) If no one I care for ever cares for me, which is very unlikely, I can still find enjoyment in friendships, in work, in books, and in other things.
d) If someone I deeply care for rejects me, that will be most unfortunate; but I will hardly die!
e) Even though I have not had much luck in winning great love in the past, that hardly proves that I *must* gain it now.
f) No evidence exists for *any* absolutistic *must*. Consequently, no proof exists that I must always have *anything*, including love.
g) Many people exist in the world who never get the kind of love they crave and who still lead happy lives.
h) At times during my life I know that I have remained unloved and happy; so I most probably can feel happy again under unloving conditions.

i) If I get rejected by someone for whom I truly care, that may mean that I possess some poor, unloving traits. But that hardly means that I am a rotten, worthless, totally unlovable individual.

j) Even if I had such poor traits that no one could ever love me, I would still not have to down myself as a lowly, bad individual.

4. DOES ANY EVIDENCE EXIST OF THE TRUTH OF THIS BELIEF?
ILLUSTRATIVE ANSWER:
No, not really. Considerable evidence exists that if I love someone dearly and never am loved in return that I will then find myself disadvantaged, inconvenienced, frustrated, and deprived. I certainly would prefer, therefore, not to get rejected. But no amount of inconvenience amounts to a *horror*. I can still *stand* frustration and loneliness. They hardly make the world *awful*. Nor does rejection make me a turd! Clearly, then, no evidence exists that I *must* receive love from someone for whom I really care.

5. WHAT ARE THE WORST THINGS THAT COULD *ACTUALLY* HAPPEN TO ME IF I DON'T GET WHAT I THINK I MUST (OR DO GET WHAT I THINK I MUST NOT GET)?
ILLUSTRATIVE ANSWER: If I don't get the love I think I must receive:

a) I would get deprived of various possible pleasures and conveniences.

b) I would feel inconvenienced by having to keep looking for love elsewhere.

c) I might *never* gain the love I want, and thereby continue indefinitely to feel deprived and disadvantaged.

d) Other people might down me and consider me pretty worthless for

getting rejected – and that would be annoying and unpleasant.

e) I might settle for pleasures other than and worse than those I could receive in a good love relationship; and I would find that distinctly undesirable.

f) I might remain alone much of the time; which again would be unpleasant.

g) Various other kinds of misfortunes and deprivations might occur in my life – none of which I need define as *awful, terrible*, or *unbearable*.

6. WHAT GOOD THINGS COULD I MAKE HAPPEN IF I DON'T GET WHAT I THINK I MUST (OR DO GET WHAT I THINK I MUST NOT GET)?

a) If the person I truly care of does not return my love, I could devote more time and energy to winning some-else's love – and probably find someone better for me.

b) I could devote myself to other enjoyable pursuits that have little to do with loving or relating, such as work or artistic endeavors.

c) I could find it challenging and enjoyable to teach myself to live happily without love.

d) I could work at achieving a philosophy of fully accepting myself even when I do not get the love I crave.

You can take any one of your major irrational beliefs – your *shoulds, oughts,* or *musts* – and spend at least ten minutes every day, often for a period of several weeks, actively and vigorously disputing this belief. To help keep yourself devoting this amount of time to the DIBS method of rational disputing, you may use operant conditioning or self-management methods (originated by B.F. Skinner, David Premack, Marvin Goldfried, and other psychologists). Select some activity that you highly enjoy that you tend to do every day – such as reading, eating, television viewing, exercising, or social contact with friends. Use this activity as a reinforcer or reward by ONLY allowing yourself to engage in it AFTER you have practiced Disputing Irrational Beliefs (DIBS) for at least ten minutes that day. Otherwise, no reward!

In addition, you may penalize yourself every single day you do NOT use DIBS for at least ten minutes. How? By making yourself perform some activity you find distinctly unpleasant – such as eating something obnoxious, contributing to a cause you hate, getting up a half-hour earlier in the morning, or spending an hour conversing with someone you find boring. You can also arrange with some person or group to monitor you and help you actually carry out the penalties and lack of rewards you set for youself. You may of course steadily use DIBS without any self-reinforcement, since it becomes reinforcing in its own right after a while. But you may find it more effective at times if you use it along with rewards and penalties that you execute immediately after you practice or avoid practicing this rational-emotive method.

Summary of Questions to Ask Yourself in DIBS

1. WHAT SELF-DEFEATING IRRATIONAL BELIEF DO I WANT TO DISPUTE AND SURRENDER?
2. CAN I RATIONALLY SUPPORT THIS BELIEF?
3. WHAT EVIDENCE EXISTS OF THE *FALSENESS* OF THIS BELIEF?
4. DOES ANY EVIDENCE EXIST OF THE *TRUTH* OF THIS BELIEF?
5. WHAT ARE THE WORST THINGS THAT COULD *ACTUALLY* HAPPEN TO ME IF I DON'T GET WHAT I THINK I MUST (OR DO GET WHAT I THINK I MUST NOT GET)?
6. WHAT GOOD THINGS COULD I MAKE HAPPEN IF I DON'T GET WHAT I THINK I MUST (OR DO GET WHAT I THINK I MUST NOT GET)?

Disputing (D) your dysfunctional or irrational Beliefs (iBs) is one of the most effective of REBT techniques. But it is still often ineffective, because you can easily and very strongly hold on to an iB (such as, 'I *absolutely must* be loved by so-and-so, and it's *awful* and I am an *inadequate person* when he/she does not love me!'). When you question and challenge this iB you often can come up with an Effective New Philosophy (E) that is accurate but weak: 'I guess that there is no reason why so-and-so *must* love me, because there are other people who will love me when so-and-so does not. I can therefore be reasonably happy without his/her love.' Believing this *almost* Effective New Philosophy, and believing it *lightly*, you can still *easily* and *forcefully* believe, 'Even though it is not awful and terrible when so-and-so does not love me, it really *is*! No matter what, I still *need* his/her affection!'

Weak, or even moderately strong, Disputing will therefore often not work very *well* to help you truly disbelieve some of your powerful and long-held iBs; while vigorous, persistent Disputing is more likely to work.

One way to do highly powerful, vigorous Disputing is to use a tape recorder and to state one of your strong irrational Beliefs into it, such as, 'If I fail this job interview I am about to have, that will prove that I'll never get a good job and that I might as well apply only for low-level positions!'

Figure out several Disputes to this iB and *strongly* present them on this same tape. For example: 'Even if I do poorly on this interview, that will only show that I failed this time, but will never show that I'll *always* fail and can *never* do well in other interviews. Maybe they'll *still* hire me for the job. But if they don't, I can learn by my mistakes, can do better in *other* interviews, and can finally get the kind of job that I want.'

Listen to your Disputing on tape. Let other people, including your therapist or members of your therapy group, listen to it. Do it over in a more forceful and vigorous manner and let them listen to it again, to see if you are disputing more forcefully, until they agree that you are getting better at doing it. Keep listening to it until you see that you are able to convince yourself and others that you are becoming more powerful and more convincing.

* * * * * * * * * * * * * *

Additional copies of this pamplet are available from the
INSTITUTE FOR RATIONAL-EMOTIVE THERAPY
45 East 65th Street, New York, NY 10021–6593
Tel (001) (212) 535–0822   Fax (001) (212) 249–3582

Call for ordering information.

APPENDIX 4

How to Maintain and Enhance Your Rational Emotive Behaviour Therapy Gains

Albert Ellis

If you work at using the principles and practices of rational emotive behavior therapy (REBT), you will be able to change your self-defeating thoughts, feelings, and behaviors and to feel much better than when you started therapy. Good! But you will also, at times, fall back – and sometimes far back. No one is perfect and practically all people take one step backwards to every two or three steps forward. Why? Because that is the nature of humans: to improve, to stop improving at times, and sometimes to backslide. How can you (imperfectly!) slow down your tendency to fall back? How can you maintain and enhance your therapy goals? Here are some methods that we have tested at the Institute for Rational-Emotive Therapy in New York and that many of our clients have found quite effective.

How to maintain your improvement

1. When you improve and then fall back to old feelings of anxiety, depression, or self-downing, try to remind yourself and pinpoint exactly what thoughts, feelings, and behaviors you once changed to bring about your improvement. If you again feel depressed, think back to how you previously used REBT to make yourself undepressed. For example, you may remember that:
   (a) You stopped telling yourself that you were worthless and that you couldn't ever succeed in getting what you wanted.
   (b) You did well in a job or in a love affair and proved to yourself that you did have some ability and that you were lovable.
   (c) You forced yourself to go on interviews instead of avoiding them and thereby helped yourself overcome your anxiety about them.
      Remind yourself of thoughts, feelings, and behaviors that you have changed and that you have helped yourself by changing.
2. Keep thinking, thinking and thinking rational beliefs (rBs) or coping statements, such as: 'It's great to succeed but I can fully accept myself as a person and enjoy life considerably even when I fail!' Don't merely parrot these statements but go over them carefully many times and think them through until you

really begin to believe and feel that they are true.

3. Keep seeking for, discovering, and disputing and challenging your irrational beliefs (iBs) with which you are once again upsetting yourself. Take each important irrational belief – such as, 'I have to succeed in order to be a worthwhile person!' – and keep asking yourself: 'Why is this belief true?' 'Where is the evidence that my worth to myself, and my enjoyment of living, utterly depends on my succeeding at something?' 'In what way would I be totally acceptable as a human if I failed at an important task or test?'

   Keep forcefully and persistently disputing your irrational beliefs whenever you see that you are letting them creep back again. And even when you don't actively hold them, realize that they may arise once more, bring them to your consciousness, and preventively – and vigorously! – dispute them.

4. Keep risking and doing things that you irrationally fear – such as riding in elevators, socializing, job hunting, or creative writing. Once you have partly overcome one of your irrational fears, keep acting against it on a regular basis. If you feel uncomfortable in forcing yourself to do things that you are unrealistically afraid of doing, don't allow yourself to avoid doing them – and thereby to preserve your discomfort forever! Often, make yourself as *un*comfortable as you can be, in order to eradicate your irrational fears and to become unanxious and comfortable later.

5. Try to clearly see that difference between appropriate negative feelings – such as those of sorrow, regret, and frustration, when you do not get some of the important things you want – and inappropriate negative feelings – such as those of depression, anxiety, self-hatred, and self-pity, when you are deprived of desirable goals and plagued with undesirable things. Whenever you feel over-concerned (panicked) or *unduly* miserable (depressed) acknowledge that you are having a statistically normal but a psychologically unhealthy feeling and that you are bringing it on yourself with some dogmatic *should, ought,* or *must.* Realize that you are invariably capable of changing your inappropriate (or *mus*turbatory) feelings back into appropriate (or preferential) ones. Take your depressed feelings and work on them until you *only* feel sorry and regretful. Take your anxious feelings and work on them until you *only* feel concerned and vigilant. Use rational-emotive imagery to vividly imagine unpleasant activating events before they happen; let yourself feel inappropriately upset (anxious, depressed, enraged, or self-downing) as you imagine them; then work on your feelings to change them to appropriate emotions (concern, sorrow, annoyance, or regret) as you keep imagining some of the worst things happening. Don't give up until you actually do change your feelings.

6. Avoid self-defeating procrastination. Do unpleasant tasks fast – today! If you still procrastinate, reward yourself with certain things that you enjoy – for example, eating, vacationing, reading, and socializing – only *after* you have performed the tasks that you easily avoid. If this won't work, give yourself a severe penalty – such as talking to a boring person for two hours or burning a hundred dollar bill – every time that you procrastinate.

7. Show yourself that it is an absorbing *challenge* and something of an *adventure* to maintain your emotional health and to keep yourself reasonably happy no matter what kind of misfortunes assail you. Make the uprooting of your misery one of the most important things in your life – something you are utterly determined to

steadily work at achieving. Fully acknowledge that you almost always have some *choice* about how to think, feel, and behave; and throw yourself actively into making the choice for yourself.

8. Remember – and use – the three main insights of REBT that were first outlined in *Reason and Emotion in Psychotherapy* (Ellis, 1962):

   Insight No. 1: You largely *choose* to disturb yourself about the unpleasant events of your life, although you may be encouraged to do so by external happenings and by social learning. You mainly feel the way you think. When obnoxious and frustrating things happen to you at point A (activating events), you consciously or unconsciously *select* rational beliefs (rBs) that lead you to feel sad and regretful and you also *select* irrational beliefs (iBs) that lead you to feel anxious, depressed, and self-hating.

   Insight No. 2: No matter how or when you acquired your irrational beliefs and your self-sabotaging habits, you now, in the present, *choose* to maintain them – and that is why you are *now* disturbed. Your past history and your present life conditions importantly *affect* you; but they don't *disturb* you. Your present *philosophy* is the main contributor to your *current* disturbance.

   Insight No. 3: There is no magical way for you to change your personality and your strong tendencies to needlessly upset yourself. Basic personality change requires persistent *work and practice* – yes, *work and practice* – to enable you to alter your irrational beliefs, your inappropriate feelings, and your self-destructive behaviors.

9. Steadily – and unfrantically! – look for personal pleasures and enjoyments – such as reading, entertainment, sports, hobbies, art, science, and other vital absorbing interests. Take as your major life goal not only the achievement of emotional health but also that of real enjoyment. Try to become involved in a long-term purpose, goal, or interest in which you can remain truly absorbed. For a good, happy life will give you something to live *for*; will distract you from many serious woes; and will encourage you to preserve and to improve your mental health.

10. Try to keep in touch with several other people who know something about REBT and who can help go over some of its aspects with you. Tell them about problems that you have difficulty coping with and let them know how you are using REBT to overcome these problems. See if they agree with your solutions and can suggest additional and better kinds of REBT disputing that you can use to work against your irrational beliefs.

11. Practice using REBT with some of your friends, relatives and associates who are willing to let you try to help them with it. The more often you use it with others, and are able to see what their iBs are and to try to talk them out of these self-defeating ideas, the more you will be able to understand the main principles of REBT and to use them with yourself. When you see other people act irrationally and in a disturbed manner, try to figure out – with or without talking to them about it – what their main irrational beliefs probably are and how these could be actively and vigorously disputed.

12. When you are in rational-emotive individual or group therapy try to tape record many of your sessions and listen to these carefully when you are in between sessions, so that some of the REBT ideas that you learned in therapy sink in. After therapy has ended, keep these tape recordings and play them back to your-

self from time to time, to remind you how to deal with some of your old problems or new ones that may arise.

13. Keep reading REBT writings and listening to REBT audio and audiovisual cassettes, particularly *Humanistic Pyschotherapy* (Ellis); *A Guide to Personal Happiness* (Ellis and Becker); *A New Guide to Rational Living* (Ellis and Harper); *Overcoming Procrastination* (Ellis and Knaus); *Overcoming Depression* (Hauck); and *A Rational Counseling Primer* (Young). Keep going back to the REBT reading and audiovisual material from time to time, to keep reminding yourself of some of the main rational-emotive findings and philosophies.

How to deal with backsliding

1. Accept your backsliding as normal – as something that happens to almost all people who at first improve emotionally and who then fall back. See it as part of your human fallibility. Don't feel ashamed when some of your old symptoms return; and don't think that you have to handle them entirely by yourself and that it is wrong or weak for you to seek some additional sessions of therapy and to talk to your friends about your renewed problems.

2. When you backslide look at your self-defeating *behavior* as bad and unfortunate; but work very hard at refusing to put *yourself* down for engaging in this behavior. Use the highly important REBT principle of refraining from rating *you*, your *self*, or your *being* but of measuring only your *acts*, *deeds*, and *traits*. You are always a *person who* acts well or badly – and never a *good person* nor a *bad person*. No matter how badly you fall back and bring on your old disturbances again, work at fully accepting yourself *with* this unfortunate or weak behavior – and then try, and keep trying, to change your behavior.

3. Go back to the ABCs of REBT and clearly see what you did to fall back to your old symptoms. At A (activating event), you usually experienced some failure or rejection once again. At rB (rational belief) you probably told yourself that you didn't *like* failing and didn't *want* to be rejected. If you only stayed with these rational beliefs, you would merely feel sorry, regretful, disappointed, or frustrated. But when you felt disturbed again, you probably then went on to some irrational beliefs (iBs), such as: 'I *must* not fail! It's *horrible* when I do!' 'I *have* to be accepted, and if I'm not that makes me an *unlovable worthless person*!' Then, after convincing yourself of these iBs, you felt, at C (emotional consequence) once again depressed and self-downing.

4. When you find your irrational beliefs by which you are once again disturbing yourself, just as you originally used disputing (D) to challenge and surrender them, do so again – *immediately* and *persistently*. Thus, you can ask yourself, 'Why *must* I not fail? Is it really *horrible* if I do?' And you can answer: 'There is no reason why I *must* not fail, though I can think of several reasons why it would be highly undesirable. It's not *horrible* if I do fail – only distinctly *inconvenient*.' You can also dispute your other irrational beliefs by asking yourself, 'Where is it written that I *have* to be accepted? How do I become an *unlovable*, *worthless person* if I am rejected?' And you can answer: 'I never *have to be* accepted, though

I would very much *prefer* to be. If I am rejected, that makes me, alas, a *person who* is rejected this time by this individual under these conditions, but it hardly makes me an *unlovable, worthless person* who will always be rejected by anyone for whom I really care.'

5. Keep looking for, finding, and actively and vigorously disputing your irrational beliefs which you have once again revived and that are now making you feel anxious or depressed once more. Keep doing this, over and over, until you build intellectual and emotional muscle (just as you would build physical muscle by learning how to exercise and then by *continuing* to exercise).

6. Don't fool yourself into believing that if you merely change your language you will always change your thinking. If you neurotically tell yourself, 'I *must* succeed and be approved' and you sanely change this self-statement to, 'I *prefer* to succeed and be approved,' you may still really be convinced, 'But I really *have to* do well and *have got to be* loved.' Before you stop your disputing and before you are satisfied with your answers to it (which in REBT we call E, or an effective philosophy), keep on doing it until you are *really* convinced of your rational answers and until your feelings of disturbance truly disappear. Then do the same thing many, many times – until your new E (effective philosophy) becomes hardened and habitual – which it almost always will if you keep working at arriving at it and re-instituting it.

7. Convincing yourself lightly or 'intellectually' of your new effective philosophy or rational beliefs often won't help very much or persist very long. Do so very *strongly* and *vigorously*, and do so many times. Thus, you can *powerfully* convince yourself, until you really *feel* it: 'I do not *need* what I *want*! I never *have* to succeed, no matter how greatly I *wish to* do so!' 'I *can* stand being rejected by someone I care for. It won't *kill* me – and I *still* can lead a happy life!' '*No* human is damnable and worthless – including and especially *me*!'

How to generalize from working on one emotional problem to working on other problems

1. Show yourself that your present emotional problem and the ways in which you bring it on are not unique and that virtually all emotional and behavioral difficulties are created by irrational beliefs (iBs). Whatever your iBs are, moreover, you can overcome them by strongly and persistently disputing and acting against these irrational beliefs.

2. Recognize that you tend to have three major kinds of irrational beliefs that lead you to disturb yourself and that the emotional and behavioral problems that you want to relieve fall into one of these three categories:
   (a) 'I *must* do well and *have* to be approved by people whom I find important.' This iB leads you to feel anxious, depressed, and self-hating; and to avoid doing things at which you may fail and avoiding relationships that may not turn out well.
   (b) 'Other people *must* treat me fairly and nicely!' This iB contributes to your feeling angry, furious, violent, and over-rebellious.
   (c) 'The conditions under which I live *must* be comfortable and free from major

hassles!' This iB tends to create your feelings of low frustration tolerance and self-pity; and sometimes those of anger and depression.

3. Recognize that when you employ one of these three absolutistic *musts* – or any of the innumerable variations on it that you can easily slide into – you naturally and commonly derive from them other irrational conclusions, such as:

 (a) 'Because I am not doing as well as I *must*, I am an incompetent worthless individual!' (Self-damnation).

 (b) 'Since I am not being approved by people whom I find important, as I *have to be*, it's *awful* and *terrible*!' (Awfulizing).

 (c) 'Because others are not treating me as fairly as nicely as they *absolutely should* treat me, they are *utterly rotten people* and deserve to be damned!' (Other-damnation).

 (d) 'Since the conditions under which I live are not that comfortable and since my life has several major hassles, as it *must* not have, I can't stand it! My existence is a horror!' (Can't-stand-it-itis).

 (e) 'Because I have failed and got rejected as I *absolutely ought not* have done, I'll *always* fail and *never* get accepted as I *must* be! My life will be hopeless and joyless forever!' (Overgeneralizing).

4. Work at seeing that these irrational beliefs are part of your *general* repertoire of thoughts and feelings and that you bring them to many different kinds of situations that are against your desires. Realize that in just about all cases where you feel seriously upset and act in a distinctly self-defeating manner you are consciously or unconsciously sneaking in one or more of these iBs. Consequently, if you get rid of them in one area and are still emotionally disturbed about something else, you can always use the same REBT principles to discover your iBs in the new area and to eliminate them there.

5. Repeatedly show yourself that it is almost impossible to disturb yourself and to remain disturbed in *any* way if you abandon your absolutistic, dogmatic *shoulds*, *oughts*, and *musts* and consistently replace them with flexible and unrigid (though still strong) *desires* and *preferences*.

6. Continue to acknowledge that you can change your irrational beliefs (iBs) by rigorously (not rigidly!) using the scientific method. With scientific thinking, you can show yourself that your irrational beliefs are only theories or hypotheses – not facts. You can logically and realistically dispute them in many ways, such as these:

 (a) You can show yourself that your iBs are self-defeating – that they interfere with your goals and your happiness. For if you firmly convince yourself, 'I *must* succeed at important tasks and *have* to be approved by all the significant people in my life,' you will of course at times fail and be disapproved – and thereby inevitably make yourself anxious and depressed instead of sorry and frustrated.

 (b) Your irrational beliefs do not conform to reality – and especially do not conform to the facts of human fallibility. If you always *had* to succeed, if the universe commanded that you *must* do so, you obviously *would* always succeed. And of course you often don't! If you invariably *had* to be approved by others, you could never be disapproved. But obviously you frequently are! The universe is clearly not arranged so that you will always get what you demand. So although your desires are often realistic, your godlike commands definitely are not!

(c) Your irrational beliefs are illogical, inconsistent, or contradictory. No matter how much you *want* to succeed and to be approved, it never follows that therefore you *must* do well in these (or any other) respects. No matter how desirable justice or politeness is, it never *has to* exist.

Although the scientific method is not infallible or sacred, it efficiently helps you to discover which of your beliefs are irrational and self-defeating and how to use factual evidence and logical thinking to rid yourself of them. If you keep using scientific analysis, you will avoid dogma and set up your hypotheses about you, other people, and the world around you so that you always keep them open to change.

7. Try to set up some main goals and purposes in life – goals that you would like very much to reach but that you never tell yourself that you absolutely must attain. Keep checking to see how you are coming along with these goals; at times revise them; see how you feel about achieving them; and keep yourself goal-oriented for the rest of your days.

8. If you get bogged down and begin to lead a life that seems too miserable or dull, review the points made in this pamphlet and work at using them. Once again: if you fall back or fail to go forward at the pace you prefer, don't hesitate to return to therapy for some booster sessions.

APPENDIX 5

Workplace Problem (A)	Self-Defeating Beliefs (B)	Emotional/ Behavioural Consequences (C)	Disputing Self-Defeating Beliefs (D)	New Effective Approach to Problem (E)

An Introduction to Rational Emotive Behaviour Therapy

Michael Neenan

Rational Emotive Behaviour Therapy (REBT) was founded in 1955 by an American psychologist, Albert Ellis. Ellis believed, like some ancient philosophers, that it is not so much events, circumstances or other people that directly cause our emotional problems but rather our beliefs and attitudes about these situations that largely determine how we think and feel. For example, three people lose their jobs: the first becomes depressed because he believes he is now worthless; the second becomes angry because he believes he should have been promoted rather than sacked; the third is happy because he never liked the job and can now pursue new opportunities. The same event for each person but three very different emotional reactions; in each case, it is the individual's beliefs about losing his job that primarily shapes his emotional response.

Ellis has identified two kinds of beliefs which are at the core of our emotional responses to various situations. The first kind are rational beliefs which are flexible and adaptable to life events. These beliefs come in the form of wishes, wants, hopes, preferences, desires. Rational beliefs are seen as logical, realistic, practical, goal-orientated and encourage the individual to strive for a philosophy of self-acceptance as a fallible human being.

The second kind are irrational beliefs which are inflexible and dogmatic and come in the form of absolute musts, shoulds, have tos, got tos, oughts – demands and commands we make on ourselves, others and the world and, when not met, can lead to 'awful' consequences (the imagined worst that could happen to us) including self-damnation and self-rejection. Irrational beliefs are seen as illogical, unrealistic and bring undesirable practical consequences; in effect, they cause considerable emotional unhappiness and can block us from achieving our goals in life.

In REBT, irrational beliefs are targeted for disputing in order to reduce or remove an individual's emotional disturbance (as will be described later, only certain kinds of negative emotional states are seen as unhealthy or self-defeating). REBT provides a model, ABC, to show how this is achieved by emphasizing the relationship between beliefs and emotions.

A	Activating Event	Giving a speech to a group of people.
B	Beliefs (Irrational)	I must not make mistakes or bore people.
		If I give a poor speech, I will be a complete failure.
		People will laugh at me and that would be awful.
		I couldn't bear to be despised or ridiculed.
C	Consequences:	
	Emotion	Anxiety
	Behaviour	Visible agitation and lack of concentration on the speech.

From the REBT viewpoint, B not A primarily causes C. Beliefs are not treated as facts but as assumptions which can be shown, to varying degrees, to be true or false and therefore open to challenge and change. The client is encouraged to weigh the evidence for and against her beliefs. The aim is to construct through disputing (D) a rational and effective (E) belief system not only to tackle the problems brought to therapy, but also to achieve a more profound philosophical change in her life (if the latter goal is sought by the client).

In order to test the effectiveness of the new rational beliefs, client and therapist negotiate which tasks or homework assignments the client will carry out between therapy sessions. These tasks enable clients to develop greater confidence and responsibility in facing their problems as well as demonstrating that what happens outside of therapy is more important than what happens inside it. With the ABC example, the client's task would be to give another speech in order to challenge her irrational or self-defeating beliefs.

A	Activating Event	Giving a speech to a group of people
B	Beliefs (Rational)	I sincerely hope I do not make mistakes or bore people but there is no reason why I absolutely must not do so. If I do, too bad.
		If I give a poor speech it means I've failed in this particular area but it doesn't mean I'm a failure as a person. I can still accept myself for failing and learn how to deliver a better speech.
		If people did laugh at me it might be difficult to cope with but hardly awful. It's me that's introducing the horror into an unpleasant situation.
		I certainly wouldn't like to be despised but I could bear it. Public ridicule may well give me a chance to strengthen my self-acceptance as well as increase my ability to tolerate uncomfortable situations.
C	Consequences:	
	Emotion	Concern
	Behaviour	More relaxed and focused on the speech.

In the above example, if the client sticks with her rational beliefs and thereby makes herself only concerned, not anxious, she is more likely to give a good speech rather than a poor one.

With regard to feelings, REBT does not aim to eliminate all emotional states — thinking, feeling and behaving constructively are equally important; instead, REBT seeks to distinguish between unhealthy and healthy negative emotions. Unhealthy negative emotions such as anxiety, depression, guilt, anger, shame, hurt, cause considerable emotional distress and produce self-defeating behaviour which blocks us from achieving our goals. Irrational beliefs create unhealthy emotions.

Healthy negative emotions and alternatives to those just listed are, respectively, concern, sadness, remorse, annoyance, regret, disappointment and, whilst signalling some degree of emotional upset, act as a stimulus to tackle self-defeating behaviour in order to reach our goals. Rational beliefs produce healthy emotions.

As can be seen from this introduction, REBT expects clients to work hard to identify, challenge and change their irrational beliefs and carry out homework tasks. Because of this emphasis, REBT employs a collaborative relationship between client and therapist. The ultimate aim of therapy is for the client to learn the principles and practices of REBT for present and future problem solving; in essence, to become his or her own counsellor.

Author's note:
The purpose of the Introduction is to provide a handout for clients, students, trainers and any other interested parties. In the ABC example, I have deliberately avoided teasing out the clinically relevant part of the A (also known as the Critical A) in order to keep the introduction relatively straightforward. Please do not disturb yourselves about my lack of theoretical purity.

APPENDIX 7

Stress Mapping

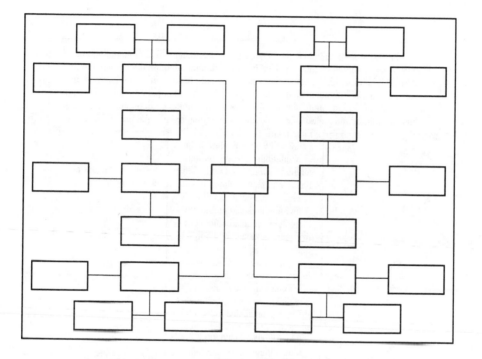

A stress map is a visual means of representing the sources of stress in your life. The central box represents yourself and the other boxes represent people you are in contact with. The other boxes can represent other potential stressors, too, such as new computers or internal demands you place on yourself, e.g. perfectionist beliefs.

Complete the boxes and then rate the amount of stress each other potential stressor can cause you on a scale of 1 to 10, where 10 represents high levels of stress. Place the score next to the appropriate stressor. Then ask yourself how much stress you may cause the other people on your stress map. Also note these scores down.

Once the exercise is completed, note down any insights that you may have gained from undertaking stress mapping.

Source: Palmer, 1990

Big I/Little i Diagram

SELF

particular action
or trait

Source: Lazarus (1977)

APPENDIX 9
Irrational Belief: Cost-benefit Form

Irrational Belief: ....

....

....

Advantages	Disadvantages

N.B. An irrational belief consists of a rigid and unqualified must, should, have to, got to, ought and a derivative which is usually awfulizing, I-can't-stand-it-itis (LFT) or damnation of self and/or others.

APPENDIX 10
Rational Belief: Cost-benefit Form

Rational Belief: ....

....

....

Advantages	Disadvantages

N.B. A rational belief consists of a flexible preference, wish, want, desire and a derivative which is usually de-awfulizing, I can stand it (HFT) or acceptance of self and/or others.

Index

Page numbers in **bold** indicate major treatment of a subject